高等职业教育教材

实用药学英语

高小丽　主编

赵文婷　杨小超　副主编

化学工业出版社

·北京·

内容简介

《实用药学英语》分为 3 个模块。模块 1　药学通用知识，主要包括人体健康、疾病、药品分类及应用等基础内容。模块 2　药品生产，包括药品生产规范、药品生产流程、药品质量检测。模块 3　药品经营与管理，包括药品说明书、药品销售、药品管理内容。3 个模块细分为 10 个单元和 3 个综合训练 (Mini Project)。每个单元内容包括 Lead-in，In-depth Reading，Extended Reading。Mini Project 包括听、说、读、写练习。

本教材适合高等职业院校药学类专业学生学习和使用，也可供药品生产、经营、管理等部门的药学工作者学习参考。

图书在版编目（CIP）数据

实用药学英语 / 高小丽主编；赵文婷，杨小超副主编. —北京：化学工业出版社，2023.6
　ISBN 978-7-122-43224-7

　Ⅰ . ①实… 　Ⅱ . ①高…②赵…③杨… 　Ⅲ . ①药物学 - 英语
Ⅳ . ① R9

中国国家版本馆 CIP 数据核字（2023）第 056344 号

责任编辑：王　芳　蔡洪伟　　　文字编辑：曹　敏
责任校对：宋　夏　　　　　　　　装帧设计：关　飞

出版发行：化学工业出版社
　　　　　（北京市东城区青年湖南街13号　邮政编码100011）
印　　装：三河市延风印装有限公司
787mm×1092mm　1/16　印张6¾　字数130千字
2023年9月北京第1版第1次印刷

购书咨询：010-64518888　　　售后服务：010-64518899
网　　址：http://www.cip.com.cn

前 言

　　实用药学英语是高等职业院校药学类专业的专业基础课程。本教材在大学英语、药物制剂技术、药品市场营销、药品管理法规等课程内容基础之上，用英语介绍药品生产、经营、管理有关的基础知识和操作技能。通过本教材的学习，使学生掌握药学方面的专业英语词汇及语句，能由浅入深地阅读专业英文资料，提升专业英语应用能力。

　　本教材以学生为中心，按照药学类专业学生毕业后可能从事的工作岗位要求，将内容进行模块化、情景化设计，并在每个模块后设计了综合训练（Mini Project）。通过真实情景化的听说读写训练，将药品生产、销售和管理等岗位的实际工作融入其中，例如设置在药房环境下的药品销售情景对话、药企的药品生产流程等真实应用情景，均来自实际工作，充分体现了职业实用性。

　　本教材由重庆化工职业学院联合陆军军医大学、重庆药友制药有限责任公司共同编写，由重庆化工职业学院高小丽担任主编，重庆化工职业学院赵文婷、陆军军医大学杨小超担任副主编。具体分工为：高小丽负责编写第一单元（Unit 1 Human and Disease），杨小超负责编写第二单元（Unit 2 What Is Drug?），李佩纹负责编写第三单元（Unit 3 Drug Clarification）、第四单元（Unit 4 Drug Regulations）及综合训练一（Mini Project 1），赵文婷负责编写第五单元（Unit 5 Pharmaceutical Operation）、第六单元（Unit 6 Traditional Chinese Medicine Processing）、第七单元（Unit 7 Drugs Quality Control）及综合训练二（Mini Project 2），姚彦君负责编写第八单元（ Unit 8 Insert）、第九单元（Unit 9 Medicine Sale ）及综合训练三（Mini Project 3），刘莉萍负责编写第十单元（Unit 10 Drug Administration）。全书框架结构的策划及全书的修改定稿由高小丽完成。

　　本书由广东食品药品职业学院丁立教授主审，并提出了宝贵的建设性意见，同时也得到了重庆药友制药有限责任公司、万和医药集团等企业的支持和帮助，在此表示衷心感谢。

　　由于编者水平有限，书中疏漏之处在所难免，敬请专家、读者批评指正。

编者
2022 年 4 月

Contents

Model 1

General Knowledge of Pharmacy

Unit 1　Human and Disease

Lead-in

In 1953, the World Health Organization（WHO）put forward the slogan "Health is Gold", aiming to arouse us to cherish health and to raise awareness of self-care. In the past, people believed that only diseases were the killer of health. In fact, bad living habits are the biggest threat to health. Life cannot be overdrawn, and everyone is required to learn more about medical knowledge, and live a healthy life.

In-depth Reading

Preview question

What is a disease according to your cognition?

Text

Information about Human Health and Disease

WHO's definition of health: Health is a state of complete physical, mental and social well-being and not merely the absence of disease or infirmity.

1. What is a disease?

Then what is a disease? It may be defined as a condition that impairs the proper function of the body or one of its parts. Every living thing, both plants and animals, can succumb to a disease. People, for example, are often infected by tiny bacteria. And bacteria can be infected by even more minute viruses.

Hundreds of different diseases exist. Each has its own particular set of symptoms and signs, clues that enable a physician to diagnose the problem. A symptom is something a patient can detect, such as fever, bleeding, or pain. A sign is something a doctor can detect, such as a swollen blood vessel or an enlarged internal body organ. Diseases can be classified differently. An acute disease has a quick onset and runs a short course. An acute heart attack, for example, often hits without warning and can be quickly fatal. A chronic disease has a slow onset and sometimes runs a years-long course. Between the acute and chronic, another type is called subacute.

2. Acute disease

Acute disease is usually characterized by the rapid onset of symptoms, short duration and severe symptoms. The symptoms often emerge abruptly and intensely, and subside quickly. Some acute diseases may not require intervention by health care professionals, such as common cold or diarrhea, because of self-treatment and use of over-the-counter medications. Some acute diseases are serious, such as acute pneumonia or appendicitis. The medical treatment for these diseases is required. Following an acute disease, most people return to their normal health status, and some become chronic disease patients.

3. Chronic disease

Chronic disease is typically characterized by a permanent change, causing or being caused by irreversible alterations in normal anatomy and physiology, requiring special health education for rehabilitation, and requiring long-term care or support. It usually lasts at least for 6 months, even for whole life process. The onset of chronic disease is slow. Symptoms are not typical or don't appear in the early stage of chronic disease.

Chronic illnesses are leading health problem in the globe. They encompass many different physical and emotional alternations in health. Arthritis, heart diseases, diabetes and hypertension are examples of chronic illness, and these diseases can't be cured. Issues of coping and living with a chronic disease are complex and overwhelming. The goal of managing a chronic illness is to control the appearance of symptoms or to improve symptoms.

Vocabulary

physical [ˈfɪzɪkl] *adj.* 身体的；物质的；物理的，物理学的

mental [ˈmentl] *adj.* 精神的，思想的；疯癫的

infirmity [ɪnˈfɜːrməti] *n.* （尤指老年的）体弱，病弱；疾病；缺点

impair [ɪmˈper] *v.* 损害，削弱

succumb [səˈkʌm] *v.* 屈服；病情加重，死于（某疾病）

bacteria [bækˈtɪriə] *n.* 细菌（bacterium 的复数）

virus [ˈvaɪrəs] *n.* 病毒；病毒性疾病；（计算机）病毒

symptom [ˈsɪmptəm] *n.* （医）症状；迹象，征兆

diagnose [ˌdaɪəgˈnoʊs] *v.* 诊断；找出原因

detect [dɪˈtekt] *v.* 查明，察觉；检测，识别

swollen [ˈswoʊlən] *adj.* 肿胀的；涨水的

vessel [ˈvesl] *n.* 船，舰；（人或动物的）血管，（植物的）导管；容器

organ [ˈɔːrgən] *n.* （人体或动植物的）器官

acute [əˈkjuːt] *adj.* 严重的，急性的，剧烈的；敏锐的，有洞察力的

fatal [ˈfeɪtl] *adj.* 致命的；导致失败的，灾难性的

chronic [ˈkrɑːnɪk] *adj.* （疾病）慢性的，长期的

onset [ˈɑːnset] *n.* （尤指某种坏事情的）开始，发作

subacute [ˌsʌbəˈkjʊt] *adj.* 亚急性的

duration [duˈreɪʃn] *n.* 持续，持续时间

emerge [ɪˈmɜːrdʒ] *v.* 浮现，出现；显露，知悉

subside [səbˈsaɪd] *v.* 趋于平静，平息；（肿）消退

intervention [ˌɪntərˈvenʃn] *n.* 干预，介入；（为改善情况尤指病痛采取的）措施

irreversible [ˌɪrɪˈvɜːrsəbl] *adj.* 不可挽回的，无法逆转的；不能治愈的

anatomy [əˈnætəmi] *n.* 解剖学；（动植物的）解剖构造；剖析

rehabilitation [ˌriːəˌbɪlɪˈteɪʃn] *n.* 康复，复原；（名誉的）恢复

arthritis [ɑːrˈθraɪtɪs] *n.* 关节炎

diabetes [ˌdaɪəˈbiːtiːz] *n.* 糖尿病，多尿症

hypertension [ˌhaɪpərˈtenʃn] *n.* 高血压；过度紧张

overwhelming [ˌoʊvərˈwelmɪŋ] *adj.* 难以抗拒的；巨大的，压倒性的

diminish [dɪˈmɪnɪʃ] *v.* 减弱，降低；贬低，轻视

tolerance [ˈtɑːlərəns] *n.* 忍受，容忍；忍耐力；耐药力，耐受性

Notes

WHO

世界卫生组织（World Health Organization，WHO）简称世卫组织，是联合国下属的一个专门机构，总部设置在瑞士日内瓦，是国际上最大的政府间卫生组织，其宗旨是使全世界人民获得尽可能高水平的健康。世界卫生组织的主要职能包括：促进流行病和地方病的防治；提供和改进公共卫生、疾病医疗和有关事项的教学与训练；推动制定生物制品的国际标准。

Translation

人类健康及疾病

世界卫生组织对健康的定义是：健康是一种生理、心理、社会适应均良好的状态，而不仅仅是指没有疾病或体质健壮。

1. 什么是疾病？

疾病可以被定义为损害身体或其中一部分的正常功能的生理状况。不管是植物还是动物，每一种生物都可能患有疾病。例如，人们经常被微小的细菌感染而患病。同时，细菌又可以被更微小的病毒感染。

疾病种类很多。每种疾病都有其特定的症状和体征，这使医生能够诊断出具体的问题。症状是患者可以感受到的，例如发烧、出血或疼痛，而体征是医生可以检测到的，例如血管的肿胀或内脏的肿大。疾病可以有不同的分类：急性疾病起病快，病程短。例如，急性心脏病经常在没有预兆的情况下发作，并且很快就会致死。慢性病起病慢，有时病程长达数年。而在急性和慢性之间，还有另一种类型称为亚急性。

2. 急性疾病

急性疾病通常以症状出现迅速、持续时间短和症状严重为特征。急性疾病的症状通常出现得很突然，表现得很强烈，然后很快消退。一些急性疾病可能不需要专业医疗人员的干预，比如普通感冒或腹泻，因为患者会自行处理或者使用非处方药。而一些严重的急性疾病，需要进行治疗，比如急性肺炎或急性阑尾炎。在经历急性疾病之后，大多数人会恢复正常的健康状态，而有些人会成为慢性疾病患者。

3. 慢性疾病

慢性疾病的典型特征是永久性的改变，它会导致解剖结构和生理学上的不可逆改变，或者病症就是由这些改变引起的。慢性疾病需要专门的康复过程，并且需要长期的护理或医疗支持。慢性疾病通常会至少持续 6 个月，甚至会伴随终生。慢性疾病的起病缓慢，其症状不甚典型或在慢性疾病的早期并不出现。

慢性疾病是影响人类健康的主要问题，其包括许多不同的身体和情绪变化。关节炎、心脏病、糖尿病和高血压都是慢性病的例子，这些疾病是无法被完全治愈的。慢性疾病的治疗是任重而道远的。慢性疾病的治疗目标是控制或缓解病症。

Quiz

Ⅰ. Answer the questions according to the text.

1. What is the definition of health and disease?

_____

2. What is the difference between a symptom and a sign?

_____

3. Can acute disease and chronic disease be transformed into each other?

_____

4. What is the goal of managing a chronic disease?

_____

Ⅱ. Complete the sentences with the words given. Change the form if necessary.

detect	acute	infect	definition
typically	medication	mental	fatal

1. Sherlock Holmes is a famous _____ in stories.

2. The _____ injuries for swimmers were muscular chronic injuries at spine region.

3. The differences between manual labor and _____ labor are diminishing in some developed countries.

4. The _____ should ease the suffering.

5. These are places for _____ trauma and treatable illness.

6. Density is _____ as mass divided by volume.

7. When viruses _____ a cell, they inject their DNA.

8. Without treatment, many of these diseases can be _____.

Ⅲ. Translation between English and Chinese.

succumb to a disease	chronic illness
swollen blood vessel	irreversible alterations
急性疾病	身心的
健康问题	内脏

Extended Reading

Text

COVID-19

1. What is COVID-19?

Corona virus disease 2019, COVID-19, is the disease caused by an infection of the SARS-CoV-2 virus. COVID-19 has spread around the world, causing unprecedented levels of illness and deaths.

The SARS-CoV-2 virus is from the family of viruses called coronaviruses that usually causes respiratory tract infection. There are multiple variants of the virus including Alpha, Beta, Gamma, Delta and Omicron, etc.

2. What are the symptoms of COVID-19?

The most common symptoms of COVID-19 include dry cough, fever, and fatigue. It is thought that symptoms can appear between 2-14 days after exposure although there have been isolated cases which suggest this may be longer.

According to the World Health Organization (WHO), symptoms of COVID-19 include: fever or chills, dry cough, fatigue, shortness of breath or difficulty breathing, sore throat, congestion or runny nose, muscle or body aches, dizziness, headache, nausea or vomiting, diarrhea, loss of taste or smell. Some people have no symptoms.

3. How do you get COVID-19?

COVID-19 is spread from one person to another when an infected person breathes out small droplets that contain virus and then the next person becomes infected when the virus enters his/her body by:breathing in the infected droplet into his/her lung or, the droplet lands directly on eyes, nose or mouth or, a droplet finds its way onto his/her hands and then he/she touches his/her eyes, nose or mouth.

4. How do you prevent COVID-19?

The most effective way to protect yourself from COVID-19 is to get the COVID-19 vaccine as soon as possible, which helps reduce the risk of severe disease, hospitalization and death. The COVID-19 vaccine helps your body develop immunity to SARS-CoV-2.

Wash your hands regularly and thoroughly with soap and water (lather for 20 seconds), or use an alcohol-based (at least 60%) hand sanitizer.

Wear a face mask in indoor places where there are high risk of COVID-19 transmission to protect yourself and others.

Practice social distancing between yourself and others (within 6 feet, or 2 meters).

Avoid contact with others who are sick or have symptoms of COVID-19.

Cover coughs and sneezes (sneeze into a tissue).

Clean and disinfect surfaces (alcohol-based disinfectants work best for corona viruses).

Vocabulary

identify [aɪˈdentɪfaɪ] *v.* 认出，识别；查明；证明（身份）；认同

unprecedented [ʌnˈpresɪdentɪd] *adj.* 前所未有的，史无前例的

respiratory [ˈrespərətɔːri] *adj.* 呼吸的

variant [ˈveriənt] *n.* 变种，变形；*adj.* 不同的，变体的

fatigue [fəˈtiːg] *n.* 疲乏，厌倦；*v.* 使疲劳，使劳累；*adj.* 疲劳的

exposure [ɪkˈspoʊʒər] *n.* 暴露；曝光，揭发；报道，宣传

ache [eɪk] *v.* 疼痛；*n.* 疼痛；（心中的）苦痛

sore [sɔːr] *adj.* 疼痛的，酸痛的；（精神）痛苦的，困扰的；*n.* 伤处，痛处

congestion [kənˈdʒestʃən] *n.* 充血，淤血；堵车

nausea [ˈnɔːziə] *n.* 恶心，呕吐感；极端的憎恶

vomit [ˈvɑːmɪt] *v.* 呕吐；喷出；*n.* 呕吐物；呕吐

diarrhea [ˌdaɪəˈriːə] *n.* 腹泻

dizziness [ˈdɪzinəs] *n.* 头晕，头昏眼花

droplet [ˈdrɑːplət] *n.* 小滴，微滴

vaccine [vækˈsiːn] *n.* 疫苗；（计算机）杀毒软件；*adj.* 疫苗的

immunity [ɪˈmjuːnəti] *n.* 免疫力；免除，豁免

alcohol [ˈælkəhɔːl] *n.* 酒精，乙醇；醇；含酒精饮品，酒

sanitizer [ˈsænəˌtaɪzər] *n.* 消毒杀菌剂；食品防腐剂

transmission [trænzˈmɪʃn] *n.* 传递，传播，传染；（无线信号的）播送，发送

sneeze [sniːz] *v.* /*n.* 打喷嚏

alcohol-based disinfectant 含酒精的消毒液

Translation

COVID-19

1. 什么是 COVID-19？

新型冠状病毒肺炎（COVID-19）是由 SARS-CoV-2 病毒感染引起的疾病。COVID-19 在全世界范围内传播，造成了前所未有的病痛和死亡。

SARS-CoV-2 病毒来自冠状病毒家族，它们通常会引起呼吸道感染。这种病毒有多种变体，包括 Alpha、Beta、Gamma、Delta 和奥密克戎等。

2. COVID-19 的症状有哪些？

COVID-19 最常见的症状有干咳、发烧和疲劳。这些症状一般会在感染后的 2 ~ 14 天出现，个别病例时间可能会更长。根据世界卫生组织的报告，COVID-19 的症状包括：发烧或寒战；干咳；疲劳；呼吸急促或呼吸困难；咽喉痛；鼻腔充血或流鼻涕；肌肉或身体疼痛；头晕；头痛；恶心或呕吐；腹泻；个别患者出现味觉或嗅觉丧失。此外，有些患者无任何症状。

3. COVID-19 的传播途径有哪些？

当患者呼出含有病毒的飞沫后，病毒通过以下方式进入下一个人的身体进而被传染 COVID-19。

带病毒的飞沫吸入肺部；

飞沫直接落入眼睛、鼻子或嘴巴；

飞沫落到手上，然后手触摸了眼睛、鼻子或嘴巴。

4. 如何预防 COVID-19？

保护自己免受感染的最有效方法是尽快接种 COVID-19 疫苗，这有助于降低患重症、住院和死亡的风险。COVID-19 疫苗可使机体对 SARS-CoV-2 病毒产生免疫力。

定期用肥皂和水彻底洗手（起泡后持续 20 秒），或使用含有酒精（至少 60%）的洗手液洗手。

在 COVID-19 传播风险高的室内佩戴口罩，以保护自己和他人。

和他人保持社交距离（约 2 米距离）。

避免与其他生病或有 COVID-19 症状的人接触。

咳嗽和打喷嚏时注意遮掩（将喷嚏打到纸巾中）。

进行表面清洁和消毒（含酒精的消毒液对杀灭冠状病毒最有效）。

Unit 2   What Is Drug?

Lead-in

Drugs, first appeared in the early days of human society, are created in the struggle against nature. Pharmacy, like other sciences, originated from human social practice and the needs of material life. Drugs have made great contributions to the healthy development of all human beings, as well as to the reproduction and development of races.

In-depth Reading

Preview questions

1. What are the routes of absorption of drugs?
2. What is the difference between OTC and prescription drugs?

Text

What Is Drug?

A drug is any chemical substance that causes a change in an organism's physiology or psychology when consumed. Drugs are typically distinguished from food and substances that provide nutritional support. Consumption of drugs can be via inhalation, injection, ingestion, absorption via a patch on the skin, suppository, or dissolution under the tongue.

In pharmacology, a drug is a chemical substance, typically of known structure, which, when administered to a living organism, produces a biological effect. A medicinal drug, also called a medication or medicine, is a chemical substance used to treat, prevent, or diagnose a disease or to promote well-being. Traditionally drugs were obtained through extraction from medicinal plants, but more recently also by organic synthesis. Medicinal drugs may be used for a limited duration, or on a regular basis for chronic disorders.

Drugs are often classified into drug classes—groups of related drugs that have similar chemical structures, the same mechanism of action (binding to the same biological target), a related mode of action, and that are used to treat the same disease.

1. Medication

A medication or medicine is a drug taken to cure or ameliorate any symptoms of an illness or medical condition. The use may also be as preventive medicine that has future benefits but does not treat any existing or pre-existing diseases or symptoms. Dispensing of medication is often regulated by governments into three categories— over-the-counter(OTC) medicines, which are available in pharmacies and supermarkets without special restrictions; behind-the-counter medicines, which are dispensed by a pharmacist without needing a doctor's prescription; and prescription only medicines, which must be prescribed by a licensed medical professional, usually a physician. The range of medicines available without a prescription varies from country to country.

2. Recreational drug

Recreational drug use is the use of a drug (legal, controlled, or illegal) with the primary intention of altering the state of consciousness through alteration of the central nervous system in order to create positive emotions and feelings.

Some national laws prohibit the use of different recreational drugs; and medicinal drugs that have the potential for recreational use are often heavily regulated. There may be an age restriction on the consumption and purchase of legal recreational drugs. Some recreational drugs that are legal and accepted in many places include alcohol, tobacco, betel nut, and caffeine products.

Vocabulary

organism [ˈɔːrgənɪzəm] *n.* 生物，有机体

psychology [saɪˈkɑːlədʒi] *n.* 心理学；心理特点

distinguish [dɪˈstɪŋgwɪʃ] *v.* 使有别于；区别，分清

nutritional [nuˈtrɪʃənl] *adj.* 营养的

inhalation [ˌɪnhəˈleɪʃn] *n.* 吸入；吸入剂

injection [ɪnˈdʒekʃn] *n.* 注射；（液体）注入，喷入

ingestion [ɪnˈdʒestʃən] *n.* 摄取；吸收；咽下

absorption [əb'sɔːrpʃn] n. （液体、气体等的）吸收

patch [pætʃ] n. 补丁；药膏，胶布；v. 修补，缝补

suppository [sə'paːzɔːri] n. 栓剂

dissolution [ˌdɪsə'luːʃn] n. 分解，溶解

pharmacology [ˌfaːrmə'kaːlədʒi] n. 药理学

administer [əd'mɪnɪstər] v. 管理；执行，实施；给予（药物或治疗）

extraction [ɪk'strækʃn] n. 取出，提炼

synthesis ['sɪnθəsɪs] n. 综合，综合体；（化学物质的）合成

mechanism ['mekənɪzəm] n. （生物体内的）机制；机械装置；途径

ameliorate [ə'miːliəreɪt] v. 改善，减轻

dispense [dɪ'spens] v. 发放，分配；配（药），发（药）

regulate ['regjuleɪt] v. （用规则条例）控制，监管；调节，调整

pharmacy ['faːrməsi] n. 药店，（医院的）药房

pharmacist ['faːrməsɪst] n. 药剂师

prescription [prɪ'skrɪpʃn] n. 处方，药方；处方药；adj. 凭处方方可购买的

physician [fɪ'zɪʃn] n. 医生，内科医生

consciousness ['kaːnʃəsnəs] n. 知觉，清醒；意识

betel ['biːtl] n. 槟榔，槟榔叶

Notes

Consumption of drugs can be via inhalation, injection, ingestion, absorption via a patch on the skin, suppository, or dissolution under the tongue.

药物的吸收有多种方式，并与给药方式和药物剂型相关，比如气雾剂是通过吸入，注射剂是直接通过注射吸收，口服药物制剂是通过消化吸收，其他还有通过皮肤吸收，通过栓剂塞入人体腔道后吸收和舌下溶解吸收等方式。

Translation

什么是药物？

药物是任何在吸收后会引起生物体生理或心理变化的化学物质。药物通常与提供营养支持的食物和其他物质有所区别。药物的吸收可以有吸入、注射、口服、皮肤上的贴剂吸收、栓剂吸收或舌下溶解吸收等方式。

在药理学中，药物是一种化学物质，通常具有已知的结构，当给药于生物体时会产生生物效应。治疗型的药物是用于治疗、预防或诊断疾病，或者能够促进身体健康

的化学物质。传统上的药物是从药用植物中提取获得的，但近来的药物也通过有机合成来获得。药物可以在一段时间内使用，或定期用于慢性疾病。

药物通常被分成很多类别——按相似化学结构分类。按相同作用机制（与相同药物靶点结合）分类。按相关作用方式分类以及按治疗相同疾病分类。

1. 治疗型药物

治疗型药物是指为了治疗疾病，或减轻症状及改善身体状况而服用的药物。这个用途也可以是预防性的，即不是治疗现有或之前就已存在的疾病或症状，而是预防某些疾病的发生。通常将药物的配发分为三类：非处方药（乙类），药房和超市均有售，没有特别限制；非处方药（甲类），由药剂师配药，无需医生处方；以及处方药，必须由有执照的医疗专业人员（通常是医生）开具处方。无需处方即可获得的药物范围因国家和地区而异。

2. 娱乐性药物

娱乐性药物是指使用（合法、受控或非法）后通过作用中枢神经系统来改变意识状态，以产生积极的情绪和感觉的一类药物。

一些国家法律禁止使用某些娱乐性药物，同时一些具有潜在娱乐用途的治疗型药物也会受到严格监管。合法的娱乐性药物的消费和购买也可能会有年龄限制。一些娱乐性药物在很多地方是合法的、被接受的，比如酒精、烟草、槟榔和含咖啡因的产品。

Quiz

Ⅰ. Decide whether the statements are true(T) or false(F) according to the text.

1. Drugs can also be food.

2. Drugs can only be taken by mouth.

3. There are two categories of medication: over-the-counter medicines, and prescription only medicines.

4. Recreational drug includes illegal mood-altering substances like heroin, as well as everyday substances like caffeine.

Ⅱ. Complete the sentences with the words given. Change the form if necessary.

chemical   organism   consumption   extraction

license   legal   primary   administer

1. I study marine_____in their natural environment.

2. FDA stands for Food and Drug_____.

3. The soil has been poisoned with_____waste from the factory.

4. _____of oil has declined in recent years.

5. This shop is _____ to sell tobacco.

6. Hempseed oil is _____ from hempseeds.

7. She said she supports Trump for his policies on _____ immigration.

8. Intake in state _____ schools is down by 10%.

Ⅲ. Translation between English and Chinese.

provide nutritional support	有机合成
through extraction from plants	非处方药
prescription only medicines	受到严格监管
medicinal drug	化学物质

Extended Reading

Text

Common Adverse Drug Reaction

1. Overview

Every drug has adverse drug reaction. How vulnerable everybody is to these side effects depends on many different factors, which can be generally grouped as patient-related, drug-related, and environmentally or socially related. Find out if you have any characteristics that will increase your susceptibility to drug-related reactions, and what you can do to manage some of these possible side effects.

2. Risk of Developing adverse drug reaction

Every one of us is unique. However, certain individual factors make some of us more likely to develop adverse drug reaction than others. The most significant of these factors is age. The very young and the very old are ALWAYS more susceptible to unwanted reactions.

(1) Age

① Children are not small adults. The way their bodies absorb, metabolize and eliminate drugs differs from adults, and this is especially true in babies. Younger children tend to absorb medicine more slowly from the stomach but have faster intramuscular (IM) absorption rates. In early life, their liver enzymes are as immature as their kidney function. In addition, the permeability of their blood-brain barrier (restricts the passage of substances from the bloodstream to the brain) is higher.

② Older adults typically take more medicines and studies have shown they are twice as likely to go to emergency department (ED) because of an adverse drug event and seven times more likely to be hospitalized. They are more likely to be on medicines with a narrow margin between being effective or toxic such as warfarin（华法林）, insulin（胰岛素）, digoxin（地高辛）,and anti-seizure（抗癫痫）medications. Their bodies tend to have more fat and less water which may increase the duration of effect of certain drugs. In addition, metabolism in the liver and excretion through the kidneys are typically reduced. Their brains are also more sensitive to the sedating effects of drugs, and pre- existing problems, such as dizziness, eye and ear problems, may be exacerbated increasing the risk of falls.

(2) Individual factors that increase risk

① Genetics. Pharmacogenetics is the name given to the study of how genes influence reaction to drugs and genetic factors account for 20%-95% of patient variability. This field of pharmacology is rapidly evolving and testing for liver enzyme variations is becoming more widespread.

② Kidney function. If your kidneys are not functioning at full capacity, side effects are more likely to happen. Some other drugs may lose their effectiveness when kidney function is reduced.

③ Gender. Females have a lower activity of certain hepatic enzymes, a higher body fat to water ratio, and a decreased clearance of drugs through the kidneys than men. Studies have shown the incidence of drug-induced liver toxicity, gastrointestinal adverse drug reaction, and allergic skin reactions are higher in females.

(3) Drug-related factor

① The dose of the drug. The higher the dosage the greater the risk of side effects.

② The formulation used. For example, inhaled steroids directly target the lungs and produce fewer side effects than oral steroids that have more body-wide effect.

③ How the drug is absorbed, metabolized, distributed, and eliminated.

④ Other medicines that are being taken at the same time.

Vocabulary

vulnerable [ˈvʌlnərəbl] *adj.* （身体或精神）脆弱的，易受伤的；易患病的
susceptibility [sə͵septəˈbɪləti] *n.* 易受影响的特性
metabolize [məˈtæbəlaɪz] *v.* 新陈代谢
eliminate [ɪˈlɪmɪneɪt] *v.* （生理）排除，排泄；剔除；消去
stomach [ˈstʌmək] *n.* 胃；腹部

intramuscular [ˌɪntrəˈmʌskjələr] *adj.* 肌肉内的；肌肉的

enzyme [ˈenzaɪm] *n.* 酶

immature [ˌɪməˈtʃʊr] *adj.* 幼稚的，不成熟的

permeability [ˌpɜːrmiəˈbɪləti] *n.* 渗透性

margin [ˈmɑːrdʒɪn] *n.* 差额，幅度；边缘

excretion [ɪkˈskriːʃn] *n.* 排泄，排泄物；分泌，分泌物

sedate [sɪˈdeɪt] *v.* 使镇静，给……服镇静剂；*adj.* 安静的

exacerbate [ɪgˈzæsərbeɪt] *v.* 使恶化，使加剧

genetics [dʒəˈnetɪks] *n.* 遗传学；遗传特征

hepatic [hɪˈpætɪk] *adj.* 肝的

gastrointestinal [ˌgæstroʊɪnˈtestɪnl] *adj.* 胃肠的

inhale [ɪnˈheɪl] *v.* 吸入，吸气

steroid [ˈsterɔɪd] *n.* 类固醇；[有化] 甾体化合物

oral [ˈɔːrəl] *adj.* 口的，口腔的；口头的；（药物）口服的

Translation

常见的药物不良反应

1. 概述

每种药物都有不良反应。每个人对药物不良反应的敏感程度取决于许多不同的因素，这些因素通常可以分为患者因素、药物因素以及环境或社会因素。下面来了解一下您是否有会增加药物相关反应的易感性的特征，以及您可以采取哪些措施来控制其中一些可能的药物不良反应吧。

2. 药物不良反应产生的因素

我们每个人都是独一无二的。然而，某些个体因素会使药物在一些人身上产生比其他人更多的不良反应。年龄是最主要的影响因素。婴幼儿和老人更容易受到不良反应的影响。

（1）年龄

① 儿童不是缩小版的成年人，儿童的身体吸收、代谢和排泄药物的方式与成年人不同，尤其是婴幼儿。年幼的儿童胃部吸收药物慢，但肌内注射吸收快。在幼年时期，儿童的肝酶不成熟，肾功能发育也不完全。此外，儿童的血脑屏障（能阻断物质从血液进入脑组织）渗透性更高。

② 老年人通常会服用更多的药物。研究表明，由药物引起的不良事件，老年人需要急诊抢救的可能性是其他人的两倍，而住院的可能性则高达七倍。老年人更有可

能使用一些有效剂量和中毒剂量相差很小的药物，例如华法林、胰岛素、地高辛和抗癫痫药物等。老年人的身体成分往往是脂肪较多而水分较少，而这可能会增加某些药物的持续作用时间。此外，药物在肝脏中的代谢和通过肾脏的排泄通常会减少。老年人的大脑对药物的镇静作用更敏感，加上已有的如头晕、视力及听力问题，可能会加剧跌倒的风险。

（2）增加药物不良反应的机体因素

① 遗传因素。药物遗传学是研究基因如何影响人对药物的反应的，遗传因素占到患者差异性的 20% ~ 95%。这一药理学领域正在迅速发展，对肝酶变异的检测也变得越来越普遍。

② 肾脏功能。如果肾脏不能充分发挥其功能，那么服用通过肾脏代谢的药物，就更有可能产生不良反应。当肾功能下降时某些药物可能会失去效力。

③ 性别。与男性相比，女性的某些肝酶活性较低，体内脂肪与水分的比例较高，并且肾脏的药物清除率较低。研究表明，药物引起的肝毒性、胃肠道不良反应、皮肤过敏反应的发生率在女性中较高。

（3）药物相关的因素

① 药物剂量。剂量越高，其产生不良反应的风险越大。

② 给药方式。例如吸入类固醇是直接针对肺部的，而口服类固醇的全身作用更强，所以前者产生的不良反应比后者更少。

③ 药物的吸收、代谢、分布和排泄规律，即药物的药代动力学。

④ 同时服用的其他药物也对不良反应的产生有影响。

Unit 3 Drug Clarification

Lead-in

Each drug can be classified into one or more drug classes. According to the type of disease being treated, there are antibiotics, cardiovascular drugs, digestive system drugs, antineoplastic drugs, and so on. Then, what exactly is each drug class?

In-depth Reading

Preview questions

    1. What is an antibiotic?
    2. How does an antibiotic work?

Text

Antibiotics

An antibiotic is a type of active antimicrobial substance against bacteria. It is the most important type of antibacterial agent for fighting bacterial infections, and antibiotic medications are widely used in the treatment and prevention of such infections. They may either kill or inhibit the growth of bacteria. Antibiotics are not effective against viruses such as the common cold or influenza; drugs which inhibit viruses are termed antiviral drugs rather than antibiotics.

Sometimes, the term antibiotic—literally "opposing life", from the Greek roots anti, "against" and bios, "life"—is broadly used to refer to any substance used against microbes, but in the usual medical usage, antibiotics (such as penicillin) are those produced naturally (by one microorganism fighting another), whereas non-antibiotic antibacterials (such as sulfonamides) are fully synthetic. However, both classes have the same goal of killing or preventing the growth of microorganisms, and both are included in antimicrobial chemotherapy.

1. History

Antibiotics have been used since ancient times. Many civilizations used topical application of mouldy bread, with many references to its beneficial effects arising from ancient Egypt, China, Greece, and Rome. The first person to directly document the use of molds to treat infections was John Parkinson (1567—1650). Antibiotics revolutionized medicine in the 20th century. Alexander Fleming (1881—1955) discovered modern penicillin in 1928, the widespread use of which proved significantly beneficial during wartime. However, the effectiveness and easy access to antibiotics have also led to their overuse and some bacteria have evolved resistance to them. The World Health Organization has classified antimicrobial resistance as "a widespread serious threat (that) is no longer a prediction for the future, it is happening right now in every region of the world and has the potential to affect anyone, of any age, in any country".

2. How do antibiotics work?

Antibiotics work by interfering with the bacterial cell wall to prevent growth and replication of the bacteria. Human cells do not have cell walls, but many types of bacteria do, and so antibiotics can target bacteria without harming human cells.

Antibiotics are either bactericidal (they kill the bacteria) or bacteriostatic (they keep the bacteria from reproducing and growing). Antibiotics have no action on viruses that are the cause of the common cold, the flu, and many coughs, so they are not effective against these types of illnesses.

3. Classes

Antibiotics are commonly classified based on their mechanism of action, chemical structure, or spectrum of activity. Most antibiotics target bacterial functions or growth processes. Those that target the bacterial cell wall (penicillins) or the cell membrane (polymyxins, 多黏菌素类), or interfere with essential bacterial enzymes (rifamycins, 利福霉素类) have bactericidal activities. Protein synthesis inhibitors (macrolides, 大环内酯类) are usually bacteriostatic. Further categorization is based on their target specificity. Narrow-spectrum antibiotics target specific types of bacteria, such as Gram-negative or Gram-positive, whereas broad-spectrum antibiotics affect a wide range of bacteria.

Vocabulary

antibiotic [ˌæntibaɪˈɑːtɪk] *n.* 抗生素

antimicrobial [ˌæntimaɪˈkrobiəl] *adj.* 杀菌的，抗菌的；*n.* 杀菌剂，抗菌剂

influenza [ˌɪnfluˈenzə] *n.* 流行性感冒

literally [ˈlɪtərəli] *adv.* 按照字面意义地，逐字地

microbe [ˈmaɪkroʊb] *n.* 细菌，微生物

penicillin [ˌpenɪˈsɪlɪn] *n.* 青霉素

sulfonamide [sʌl ˈfɑːnəmaɪd] *n.* 磺胺类药

synthetic [sɪnˈθetɪk] *adj.* 合成的，人造的；综合的；*n.* 合成物

chemotherapy [ˌkiːmoʊˈθerəpi] *n.* [临床] 化学疗法

civilization [ˌsɪvələˈzeɪʃn] *n.* 文明；教化

mouldy [ˈmoʊldi] *adj.* 发霉的

document [ˈdɑːkjumənt] *n.* 文件；（计算机）文档；*v.* 记录，记载

replication [ˌreplɪˈkeɪʃn] *n.* 复制；回答

spectrum [ˈspektrəm] *n.* 范围，幅度；光谱，波谱

membrane [ˈmembreɪn] *n.* （动植物的）膜；膜状物

categorization [ˌkætəgərəˈzeɪʃn] *n.* 分类

specificity [ˌspesɪˈfɪsəti] *n.* [免疫] 特异性；特征；专一性

Notes

antibiotic/antibacterial/antimicrobial

抗生素（antibiotic），这个词本义是指能够干扰或抑制细菌生长的物质，但在医学中则特指由微生物或动植物所产生的具有抗病菌活性的代谢产物。抗菌剂（antibacterial agent）中既包括天然产生的抗生素，又包括人工合成的非抗生素类抗菌剂（non-antibiotic antibacterial agent）。而抗微生物剂（antimicrobial agent），不仅包含了抗菌剂，也包含了抗病毒剂（antiviral agent）等其他一些药物。

bactericidal/bacteriostatic

这两个词都是合成词。杀菌的（bactericidal），是 bacteria 加上 cidal，-cide 作为词

根是切割的意思，例如自杀（suicide）、杀菌剂（germicide）。抑菌的（bacteriostatic）是 bacteria 加上 static，static 是静止的意思，即细菌不能再生长繁殖。

Translation

抗生素

抗生素是一种对细菌有干扰或抑制作用的物质，它是抵御细菌感染的最重要的抗菌剂，抗生素药物也广泛用于治疗和预防此类感染。抗生素可以杀死细菌或者抑制细菌生长，但对普通感冒病毒或流感病毒无效，抑制病毒的药物被称为抗病毒药物而不是抗生素。

抗生素（antibiotic）这个术语——字面意思是"反对生命"，来自希腊语词根 anti，是"反对"的意思；而 bios，是"生命"的意思——广泛用于指代任何用于抵抗微生物的物质；但在医学用法中，天然抗生素（如青霉素）是自然产生的（由一种微生物对抗另一种时产生的），而非抗生素类的抗菌剂（如磺胺类物质）是全合成的。然而，这两类物质都有着杀死微生物或阻碍微生物生长的相同作用，并且都被应用于抗微生物化学疗法中。

1. 抗生素的历史

人们自古以来就使用抗生素。许多古老的文献中提到，在古埃及、中国、希腊和罗马，将发霉的面包施用在患处产生了较好的治疗效果。据载第一个使用霉菌治疗感染的人是约翰·帕金森 (John Parkinson，1567—1650)。抗生素在 20 世纪彻底革新了医药学。亚历山大·弗莱明 (Alexander Fleming, 1881—1955) 于 1928 年发现了青霉素，其在战争时期的广泛使用被证明非常有效。然而，抗生素的有效性和易得性也导致了它们的滥用，一些细菌已经对它们产生了抗药性。世界卫生组织对抗生素耐药性的评价："抗生素耐药性不再罕见，而是一种全球性的严重威胁，现在正在世界每个地区发生，并有可能影响任何年龄、任何国家的人"。

2. 抗生素是如何发挥作用的

抗生素是通过干扰细菌细胞壁（的生成）来阻碍细菌生长和复制的。人体细胞没有细胞壁，而许多种类的细菌都有，因此抗生素可以靶向到细菌而不伤害人体细胞。

抗生素要么具有杀菌作用（杀死细菌），要么具有抑菌作用（阻止细菌繁殖和生长）。抗生素对引起普通感冒、流感和咳嗽的病毒不起作用，因此对这些类型的疾病无效。

3. 抗生素的分类

通常根据抗生素的作用机制、化学结构或抗菌谱进行分类。大多数抗生素针对的是细菌的功能或生长过程。有的通过抑制细菌细胞壁（如青霉素）或细胞膜（如多黏菌素）的合成，或干扰细菌中关键酶（如利福霉素）的合成而发挥杀菌的活性。蛋白质合成抑制剂（如大环内酯类）通常具有抑制细菌生长的活性。抗生素的进一步分类则是基于它们的目标特异性。窄谱抗生素针对的是特定类型的细菌，例如革兰氏阴性菌或革兰氏阳性菌，而广谱抗生素则能够抵抗大部分的细菌。

Quiz

Ⅰ. Decide whether the statements are true(T) or false(F) according to the text.

1. Antibiotics are effective against both bacteria and viruses.

2. John Parkinson was the first person who used molds to treat infections.

3. Human cells have no cell membrane and are not harmed by antibiotics.

4. Broad-spectrum antibiotics affect more bacterial species than narrow-spectrum antibiotics.

Ⅱ. Complete the sentences with the words given. Change the form if necessary.

| bacteria | synthetic | term | document |
| interfere | specificity | function | significantly |

1. Penicillin destroys many types of bacteria by disrupting _____ of their cell walls.

2. Fortunately, his head injuries left his bodily _____ unimpaired.

3. The whole banking scandal came into the open after somebody found some confidential _____.

4. Don't _____ with him. He's preparing for the final exams.

5. Ultraviolet rays kill _____ on their feathers.

6. Trees can have a _____ impact on our cities.

7. Are you familiar with the _____ psychosis?

8. Israel hasn't really _____ what it's going to do.

Ⅲ. Translation between English and Chinese.

inhibit the growth of bacteria   since ancient times

antimicrobial resistance   cell membrane

抗菌活性   作用机制

广谱抗生素   细菌的复制

Extended Reading

Text

Nonsteroidal Anti-inflammatory Drugs

Nonsteroidal anti-inflammatory drugs (usually abbreviated to NSAIDs) are a group of medicines that relieve pain and fever and reduce inflammation.

NSAIDs all work in the same way, and that is by blocking a specific group of enzymes called cyclo-oxygenase enzymes, often abbreviated to COX enzymes. These enzymes are responsible for the production of prostaglandins. Prostaglandins are a group of compounds with hormone-like effects that control many different processes such as inflammation, blood flow, and the formation of blood clots.

1. What are NSAIDs used for?

NSAIDs are used to treat mild-to-moderate pain that arises from a wide range of conditions such as headaches, menstruation, arthritis, and toothache.

Aspirin is a NSAID that is used in small doses to lower the risks of having a heart attack or a stroke caused by a blood clot. It may also be given as a single dose at the time of a heart attack to improve outcomes.

2. What are the differences between NSAIDs?

NSAIDs may be grouped according to their preference for COX-1 and COX-2 enzymes. Most NSAIDs inhibit both enzymes to a certain extent. Those that favor COX-1 are more likely to cause gastrointestinal side effects. Those that favor COX-2 have a higher risk of cardiovascular effects but less gastrointestinal effects. Higher dosages of NSAIDs tend to result in more COX-2 enzyme inhibition (and more cardiovascular side effects), even in those NSAIDs traditionally seen as low risk (such as ibuprofen).

3. Are NSAIDs safe?

NSAIDs are one of the most widely prescribed group of medicines; however, they are associated with some serious side effects.

NSAIDs can increase the risk of a fatal heart attack or stroke. The risk increases with a high dosage and a long time you take NSAID. People with pre-existing heart disease are more likely at risk and, NSAIDs should never be used just before or after heart bypass surgery.

Gastrointestinal (GI) side effects are also common, and usually related to dosage and duration of treatment especially some NSAIDs, such as aspirin, is associated with a higher risk. Elderly people or those taking other medicines that irritate the stomach are more likely to experience life-threatening GI side effects, such as stomach or intestinal bleeding.

Most NSAIDs are not suitable for children or adolescents under the age of 18 years. Ibuprofen is the only NSAID approved for children aged three months and older.

Most NSAIDs should not be taken during the last three months of pregnancy or while breastfeeding except on a doctor's advice.

Vocabulary

nonsteroidal [ˌnɒnstəˈrɒɪdəl] *adj.* 非甾体化合物的，非类固醇的

inflammatory [ɪnˈflæmətɔːri] *adj.* 炎症性的；煽动性的

oxygenase [ˈɑːksɪdʒəˌneɪs] *n.* [生化] 加氧酶，氧合酶

abbreviate [əˈbriːvieɪt] *v.* 缩写，使省略

prostaglandin [ˌprɑːstəˈglændɪn] *n.* [生化] 前列腺素

hormone [ˈhɔːrmoʊn] *n.* 激素，荷尔蒙

clot [klɑːt] *n.* 凝块（尤指血块）；*v.* 凝结成块

menstruation [ˌmenstruˈeɪʃn] *n.* [生理] 月经，月经期间

migraine [ˈmaɪɡreɪn] *n.* 偏头痛

stroke [stroʊk] *n.* 中风；（使用武器的）击，打；击球

cardiovascular [ˌkɑːrdioʊˈvæskjələr] *adj.* 心血管的

dosage [ˈdoʊsɪdʒ] *n.* 剂量，用量

bypass [ˈbaɪpæs] *v.* 绕过；对（动脉等）做分流术；*n.* 旁路；搭桥手术

irritate [ˈɪrɪteɪt] *v.* 激怒；刺激（部位），使疼痛；使（细胞或器官）兴奋

intestinal [ˌɪnˈtestɪnəl] *adj.* 肠的

adolescent [ˌædəˈles(ə)nt] *n.* 青少年；*adj.* 青春期的

pregnancy [ˈpregnənsi] *n.* 怀孕，妊娠（期）

Translation

非甾体抗炎药

非甾体抗炎药（通常缩写为 NSAIDs）是一类具有解热、镇痛和抗炎作用的药物。

非甾体抗炎药都以相同的方式，即阻断一种特定酶组——环氧合酶来起作用，环氧合酶通常缩写为 COX 酶。这些酶负责前列腺素的产生，前列腺素是一类具有激素

样作用的化合物，它可以控制许多不同的过程，例如炎症发生、血流和血栓形成。

1. 非甾体抗炎药的用途是什么？

非甾体抗炎药用于治疗由多种原因引起的轻度至中度疼痛，例如头痛、痛经、关节疼痛和牙痛等。

阿司匹林是一种非甾体抗炎药，小剂量使用可降低因血栓引起的心脏病或中风风险，也可以在心脏病发作时单剂量给药以改善愈后。

2. 非甾体抗炎药之间的区别有哪些？

非甾体抗炎药可根据其对 COX-1 和 COX-2 酶的作用进行分类。大多数非甾体抗炎药在一定程度上对两种酶都有抑制作用。对 COX-1 酶抑制更强的药物更容易引起胃肠道副作用。对 COX-2 酶抑制更强的药物有诱发心血管疾病的风险，但对胃肠道影响较小。较高剂量的非甾体抗炎药往往会引起更强的 COX-2 酶抑制（以及更大的心血管副作用），即使那些通常被视为低风险的非甾体抗炎药（如布洛芬）也是如此。

3. 非甾体抗炎药安全吗？

非甾体抗炎药是应用最广的药物之一，然而，它们仍然与一些严重的副作用有关。

非甾体抗炎药会增加心脏病或中风的发病风险。使用剂量越高，用药时间越长，风险就越大。对于既往患有心脏病的人这种风险会更大，所以绝不能在心脏搭桥手术前后使用非甾体抗炎药。

非甾体抗炎药的胃肠道副作用也很常见，通常与用药剂量和持续用药时间有关，某些非甾体抗炎药（例如阿司匹林）风险更高。老年人或在服用其他刺激胃部药物的患者更容易出现危及生命的胃肠道副作用，比如胃肠道出血。

大多数非甾体抗炎药不适合儿童或 18 岁以下的青少年。布洛芬是唯一被批准可用于三个月以上儿童的非甾体抗炎药。

除非有医生的医嘱，大多数非甾体抗炎药都不应在孕期的最后三个月或哺乳期使用。

Mini Project 1

Section I Listening

Mini Project 1

A nurse and a student is talking about body temperature. Listen carefully, and complete Task 1.

Task 1

1. What is the normal temperature of the human body?

A. 36.5℃   B. 37℃   C. 37.3℃

2. Which is the highest, the rectal, the mouth, or the axillary temperature?

A. The rectal temperature.

B. The mouth temperature.

C. The axillary temperature.

3. Why is rectal temperature the standard?

A. Because it is the hardest to monitor.

B. Because it is the easiest to monitor.

C. Because it is close to the temperature of the blood.

4. When do we take temperature for feverish patients?

A. Every eight or four hours.

B. Every four or two hours.

C. At 8 a.m. and 4 p.m.

5. When a patient swallows mercury, which of the following is wrong?

A. Asking the patient to take some egg white.

B. Asking the patient to drink some milk.

C. Asking the patient to drink some water.

Vocabulary

rectal [ˈrektəl] *adj.* 直肠的

axillary [æk ˈsɪləri] *adj.* 腋窝的

feverish [ˈfiːvərɪʃ] *adj.* 发烧的，发热的

respiration [ˌrespəˈreɪʃn] *n.* 呼吸；（医）一次呼吸

thermometer [θərˈmɑːmɪtər] *n.* 温度计，体温计

mercury [ˈmɜːrkjəri] *n.* 汞，水银

Section II Speaking

Task 2

You are required to talk about the illustration in 3 minutes, giving your understanding of the information of the drug in the illustration.

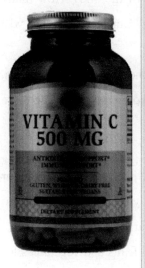

12 HEALTH BENEFITS OF VITAMIN C

1. POWERFUL ANTIOXIDANT AND PROTECTOR OF THE CELLS AND DNA
2. KEY FACTORS IN THE SYNTHESIS OF COLLAGEN
3. MAY HAVE ANTI-AGING EFFECTS
4. MAY PREVENT AND ALLEVIATE DIVERSE INFECTIONS AND COMMON COLD
5. MAY BOOST THE IMMUNE SYSTEM
6. MAY REDUCE BLOOD PRESSURE
7. MAY LESSEN THE RISK OF HEART DISEASE
8. MAY HELP PREVENT IRON DEFICIENCY ANEMIA
9. MAY IMPROVE THE HEALING OF PRESSURE ULCERS
10. MIGHT PROTECT AGAINST COGNITIVE IMPAIRMENT AND ALZHEIMER DISEASE
11. MAY IMPROVE MOOD
12. MAY LOWER LDL CHOLESTEROL (BAD CHOLESTEROL)

- ascorbic acid
- health care product
- deficiency
- nutritional
- antioxidation

Section III Reading

How to Live a Longer Life

Generally speaking, living a longer life is a good thing if you are healthy enough to enjoy it.

1. Happiness for longevity

Studies which are both informal and clinical in nature find that people who are generally positive and have a good outlook on life live longer. How do you stay positive? It's very personal, so try and find your own way.

2. Lifestyle choices lead to longer life

On average smoking kills people 14 years earlier than everybody else. Smoking causes heart disease, lung cancer and other illnesses. Just eliminating or avoiding smoking will let you live longer. Alcohol is another obvious risk factor. It leads to accidents, heart disease, cancers, and the general breaking down of the body. How many alcoholics do you see that look young? Not many I would guess. Cut back and you will live a longer life.

Many other lifestyle choices promote longevity. Seat belts are one. You should use them. Accidents are still one of the leading causes of death and if you avoid them you will be more likely to live longer.

3. The longevity diet

It has become increasingly clear that your diet has a lot to do with longevity. Keep your calorie count low, and you don't have to starve yourself. Normal daily calorie intake seems to be in the 2000 range. A 30 percent less per day is probably a good start.

Other dietary considerations consist of upping the intake of all fruits and vegetables for their nutritional and disease fighting attributes, eating more beans and legumes for their fiber and protein, and greatly increasing the consumption of fish.

4. Physical activity: conducive to longer life

There are few people who live long lives stuck to a couch and not owning walking shoes. People who live longer are typically on their feet more often and working physically every day. A poor diet and lack of exercise can lead to obesity, which reduces your life expectancy by 3 to 10 years.

Task 3

Read the passage and complete the sentences with proper words.

1. How to stay _____ is a personal thing, everyone has their own way.

2. Heart disease and lung cancer can be caused by _____ .

3. You should use _____ to minimize injures in car accidents.

4. Working _____ may make people living a longer life.

Task 4

Read the passage and choose the best answer to fill in the blanks.

1. Which of the following will not harm your health? (   )

A. Smoking   B. Alcohol

C. Obesity   D. Fiber

2. Disease fighting attributes can be get in (   ).

A. Fruits   B. Beans

C. Protein   D. Chickens

3. Which of the following is not mentioned in this passage? (   )

A. Eat less to lower your calorie intake.

B. Exercise regularly to keep fit.

C. Stress can be harmful to your health.

D. Fish are healthy food.

Section Ⅳ Writing

Task 5

Suppose you are working in a children's hospital, and you will write a note for parents on the use of children's cough syrup. Here are some pictures about the product. Discuss with your classmates and write them down.

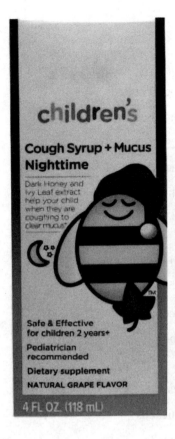

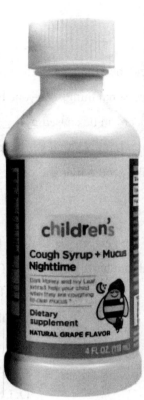

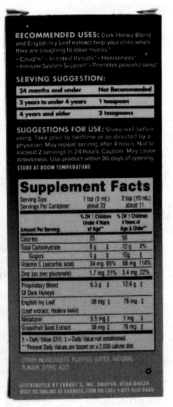

Model 2

Pharmaceutical and Quality Control

Unit 4　Drug Regulations

Lead-in

National drug standards include ChP (Chinese Pharmacopoeia), drug registration standards and other drug standards published by National Medical Products Administration(NMPA). It contains quality indicators, analytical methods and technical requirements for manufacturing. It is very important to establish standards for drugs to promote the drug administration, ensure the quality and rational use of medication, and maintain health.

In-depth Reading

Preview question

What are the objects of GMP?

Text

Good Manufacturing Practice

Good manufacturing practice (GMP) is a collection of legal technical standards for the entire drug manufacturing process. It is an effective way to provide assurance of the quality, safety and efficacy of drugs. GMP is a scientific, systemic and effective management, which can strengthen the state supervision and administration of pharmaceutical production, supervise the whole process of drugs manufacture, and guarantee quality of drugs.

Implementing GMP is to　①　minimize human error;　②　prevent the contamination of drugs and avoid the production of low-quality drugs; ③ assure the systemic design of high-quality products. The objects of GMP are ① personnel; ② environment; ③ manufacturing process. Personnel are the software of GMP, and they are also the critical object of GMP, while the other things are the hardware of GMP. Both of them are necessary.

After people suffering from the terrible drug disasters, especially the Thalidomide event which is the most infamous medical catastrophe in the 20th century, drug manufacturing quality finally drew public attention. In 1962, six professors at Temple University drafted GMP at FDA's request. In 1963, the first GMP was enforced in US, and in 1969, WHO suggested its members to carry out GMP. Since then, GMP has been implemented in over 100 countries and regions. The abbreviation of "Current Good Manufacture Practice" is cGMP.

It has been over 30 years, since GMP was first promulgated in China in 1988. GMP was revised twice in 1992 and 1998. Until June 30th, 2004, all the active pharmaceutical ingredients and preparations had been manufactured under the condition that GMP requests. On February 12th, 2011, the new edition of GMP(revised in 2010) was published, and it became effective on March 1st , 2011. The new edition of GMP is improved over the GMP 1998 edition, and the GMP published by European Union, FDA and WHO were referenced in the new edition.

Here are some articles in the 2011 GMP.

Article 38: The location, design, layout, construction, adaption and maintenance of premises should suit the drug production requirements, and should minimize the risk of contamination, cross-contamination, mixup and errors, as well as permit effective cleaning, operation and maintenance.

Article 40: The manufacturer should have a neat manufacturing environment. The ground, roads, and transportation in plant area should not introduce contamination to the manufacturing. The general layout of production, administration, living and ancillary areas should be well designed to avoid interference from each other. Premises and buildings should be well designed to ensure the logical flow of materials and personnel.

Article 42: Lighting, temperature, humidity and ventilation should be appropriate so that they do not adversely affect, directly or indirectly, either the product quality during their manufacture and storage, or the accurate functioning of equipment.

Article 43: Premises and facilities should be designed and equipped so as to afford maximum protection against the entry of insects or other animals. Necessary measures should be taken to avoid the contamination to equipment, materials and products caused by raticide, insecticide, fumigation reagent, etc.

Article 49: Interior surfaces (walls, floors and ceilings) of a clean area should be smooth, free from cracks, open joints and dust retention, should not shed particulate matter, and should permit easy and effective cleaning and, if necessary, disinfection.

Article 57: Storage areas should be of sufficient capacity to allow orderly storage of the various categories of materials and products: starting materials and packaging materials, intermediate, bulk and finished products, products in quarantine, released, rejected, returned or recalled products.

Vocabulary

pharmacopoeia [ˌfɑːrməkəˈpiːə] n. 药典

standard [ˈstændərd] n. 标准，水平，规范

registration [ˌredʒɪˈstreɪʃn] n. 登记，注册，挂号

indicator [ˈɪndɪkeɪtər] n. 标志，迹象；方向灯，转向指示灯

analytical [ˌænəˈlɪtɪkl] adj. 具备分析能力的，善于分析的；分析的，分析性的

maintain [meɪnˈteɪn] v. 保持，维持；维修，保养

efficacy [ˈefɪkəsi] n. 功效，效力

supervise [ˈsuːpərvaɪz] v. 指导工作；监督（任务、计划、活动）

implement [ˈɪmplɪment] v. 执行，贯彻；为……提供工具

contamination [kənˌtæmɪˈneɪʃn] n. 污染

personnel [ˌpɜːrsəˈnel] n. 全体人员，员工；人事部门；adj. 人员的，有关人事的

infamous [ˈɪnfəməs] adj. 声名狼藉的；无耻的

catastrophe [kəˈtæstrəfi] n. 灾难，灾祸；麻烦，困境

abbreviation [əˌbriːviˈeɪʃn] n. 缩略，缩写

promulgate [ˈprɑːmlɡeɪt] v. 发布，颁布（新法律）

layout [ˈleɪaʊt] n. 布局，设计

premise [ˈpremɪs] n. （企业或机构使用的）房屋及土地

neat [niːt] adj. 整齐的，简洁的

interference [ˌɪntərˈfɪrəns] n. 干预，干涉

humidity [hjuːˈmɪdəti] n. 潮湿，湿气；湿度

ventilation [ˌventɪˈleɪʃn] n. 通风，通风系统

appropriate [əˈproʊpriət] adj. 合适的，相称的

facility [fəˈsɪləti] n. 设施，设备

raticide [ˈrætəˌsaɪd] n. 灭鼠药

insecticide [ɪnˈsektɪsaɪd] n. 杀虫剂

fumigation [ˌfjuːmɪˈɡeɪʃn] *n.* 烟熏法；熏烟消毒法

ceiling [ˈsiːlɪŋ] *n.* 天花板，吊顶

crack [kræk] *n.* 裂缝，缝隙

retention [rɪˈtenʃn] *n.* 保持，保留；保存，存放

shed [ʃed] *v.* 掉落

sufficient [səˈfɪʃnt] *adj.* 足够的，充足的

intermediate [ˌɪntərˈmiːdiət] *adj.* 居中的，中间的

quarantine [ˈkwɔːrəntiːn] *n.* 隔离期，检疫期；隔离，检疫

Notes

Chinese Pharmacopoeia (ChP) 中华人民共和国药典

National Medical Products Administration(NMPA) 国家药品监督管理局

Good Manufacturing Practice (GMP) 药品生产质量管理规范

Thalidomide event 反应停事件　20 世纪 60 年代前后，欧美至少 15 个国家的医生都在使用沙利度胺（又名"反应停"）。这种药物可以治疗妇女妊娠反应，很多人吃了药后就不吐了，恶心的症状得到了明显改善，它成了"孕妇的理想选择"（当时的广告用语）。于是，"反应停"被大量生产、销售，仅在联邦德国就有近 100 万人服用过"反应停"，其每月的销量达到了 1 吨的水平。在联邦德国的某些州，患者甚至不需要医生处方就能购买到"反应停"。但随之而来的是，许多出生的婴儿都是短肢畸形，形同海豹，被称为"海豹畸形"婴儿。1961 年，这种症状终于被证实是孕妇服用"反应停"所导致的。于是，该药被禁用，然而，受其影响的婴儿已多达 1.2 万名。经过媒体的进一步披露，人们才发现，这起事故的产生是因为在"反应停"销售之前，有关机构并未仔细检验其可能产生的副作用。这一报道震惊了世界，引起了公众的极大愤怒，并最终迫使沙利度胺的销售者支付了赔偿。

Translation

药品生产质量管理规范

　　药品生产质量管理规范（GMP）是对药品生产全过程进行管理的法定工作技术标准。它是保证药品质量乃至用药安全的有效措施。GMP 是强化国家对药品生产的监督管理、实现对药品生产的全过程监督、保证药品质量的一套科学、系统和行之有效的管理制度。

　　推行 GMP 的目的是：①将人为造成的错误减小到最低；②防止药品的污染和低质量医药品的产生；③保证产品高质量的系统设计。GMP 管理的对象是：①人员；

②生产环境；③制剂生产的全过程。"人员"是实施 GMP 管理的软件，也是关键的管理对象，而"物"是 GMP 管理的硬件，也是必要条件，两者缺一不可。

在人类经历了多次重大的药物灾难后，特别是 20 世纪最大的药物灾难"反应停"事件，药品的生产质量引起了公众的关注。1962 年美国 FDA 组织坦普尔大学的 6 名教授编写并制定了 GMP。1963 年美国诞生了世界第一部 GMP，1969 年 WHO 建议各成员国实行 GMP 制度。至今，全球已有 100 多个国家和地区实行了 GMP 制度。cGMP 是英文"Current Good Manufacture Practice"的简称，即现行药品生产质量管理规范。

我国自 1988 年第一次颁布 GMP 至今已有 30 多年，在此期间经历 1992 年和 1998 年两次修订。截至 2004 年 6 月 30 日，实现了所有原料药和制剂均在符合 GMP 的条件下生产的目标。2011 年 2 月 12 日国家颁布了新版 GMP（2010 年修订），并于 2011 年 3 月 1 日起施行。新版 GMP 是在 1998 年版基础上更加完善的版本，在修订过程中参考借鉴了欧盟、FDA 和 WHO 的 GMP 内容。

以下是 2011 版 GMP 部分内容。

第三十八条　厂房的选址、设计、布局、建造、改造和维护必须符合药品生产要求，应当能够最大限度地避免污染、交叉污染、混淆和差错，便于清洁、操作和维护。

第四十条　企业应当有整洁的生产环境。厂区的地面、路面及运输等不应当对药品的生产造成污染。生产、行政、生活和辅助区的总体布局应当合理，不得互相妨碍。厂区和厂房内的人、物流走向应当合理。

第四十二条　厂房应当有适当的照明、温度、湿度和通风，确保生产和贮存的产品质量以及相关设备性能不会直接或间接地受到影响。

第四十三条　厂房、设施的设计和安装应当能够有效防止昆虫或其他动物进入。应当采取必要的措施，避免所使用的灭鼠药、杀虫剂、烟熏剂等对设备、物料、产品造成污染。

第四十九条　洁净区的内表面（墙壁、地面、天棚）应当平整光滑、无裂缝、接口严密、无颗粒物脱落，避免积尘，便于有效清洁，必要时应当进行消毒。

第五十七条　仓储区应当有足够的空间，确保有序存放待验、合格、不合格、退货或召回的原辅料、包装材料、中间产品、待包装产品和成品等各类物料和产品。

Quiz

I. Answer the questions according to the text.

1. What are the objects of GMP?

2. What are the requirements of the premises' location mentioned in the 2011 GMP?

_____

3. What are the requirements of interior surfaces?

_____

4. Why did WHO suggest its members to carry out GMP?

_____

Ⅱ. Complete the sentences with the words given. Change the form if necessary.

implement	humidity	maintain	quarantine
contamination	appropriate	sufficient	analytical

1. The following day she felt _____ well to go to work.

2. These plants need heat and _____ to grow well.

3. The book was written in a style _____ to the children of the age.

4. He tried to _____ a technocratic economic policy.

5. I have an _____ approach to every survey.

6. The _____ of the ocean around Puget Sound may be just the beginning.

7. She was sent home and put in _____ .

8. _____ the distance between us, make the whole team move like a whole body.

Ⅲ. Translation between English and Chinese.

GMP   中华人民共和国药典

WHO   避免药物被污染

NMPA   现行药品生产质量管理规范

packaging materials   厂房的选址

Extended Reading

Text

Good Manufacturing Practice for Drugs (2010 Revision)

Chapter 1   General provisions

Article 1: These provisions of Good Manufacturing Practice (GMP) for Drugs, in accordance with the Drug Administration Law of the People's Republic of China and the Regulations for Implementation of the Drug Administration Law of the People's

Republic of China, are enacted to regulate the manufacturing and quality management of Drugs.

Article 2: The manufacturer should establish a quality management system. The system should cover all factors that influence the quality of drugs, including all organized and planned activities with the objective of ensuring that the drugs are of the quality required for their intended use.

Article 3: GMP, as part of the quality management system, is the basic requirement of production and quality control of drugs, to ensure the products are consistently manufactured in accordance with the registration requirements, and are suitable for their intended use, by minimizing the risks of contamination, cross-contamination and mixup or errors in manufacturing process.

Article 4: The manufacturer should strictly implement GMP with integrity. Any falsification and fraud are forbidden.

Chapter 2   Quality management

Section 1   Principle

Article 5: The manufacturer should establish a quality objective to meet quality management requirements so that all registration requirements related to drug safety, efficacy and quality are systematically implemented throughout the entire process of production, control, product release, storage and distribution, to ensure that the products are manufactured in accordance with the registration requirements, and are suitable for their intended use.

Article 6: The attainment of the quality objective is the responsibility of senior management and requires the participation and commitment by staff at all levels within the manufacturer, by the manufacturer's suppliers and by the distributors.

Article 7: The manufacturer should be adequately resourced with competent personnel, suitable and sufficient premises, equipment and facilities for achieving its quality objective.

Section 3   Quality control

Article 11: Quality control is concerned with organization, documentation, sampling, testing, etc., which ensure that the necessary tests are actually carried out and materials or products are not released, until their quality has been judged to be satisfactory.

Article 12: The basic requirements of quality control are as follows.

(1) Adequate facilities, equipment, instruments and trained personnel are resourced, to ensure the related quality control activities are done effectively and reliably.

(2) Approved procedures are available for sampling, inspection, and testing starting materials, packaging materials, intermediate, bulk and finished products, and for product stability study, and where appropriate for monitoring environmental conditions, to ensure the compliance with GMP.

(3) Samples of starting materials, packaging materials, intermediate, bulk and finished products are taken by authorized personnel with approved methods.

(4) Testing methods are validated or verified.

(5) Records are made for sampling, inspecting and testing. Any deviations are investigated and recorded.

(6) The inspection and testing of materials, intermediate, bulk and finished products is formally assessed against specification, and records must be made.

…

Vocabulary

provision [prə'vɪʒn] *n.* 条款，规定

in accordance with 依照；与……一致

enact [ɪ'nækt] *v.* 制定，通过

consistently [kən'sɪstəntli] *adv.* 一贯地，始终；一致地

integrity [ɪn'tegrəti] *n.* 正直，诚实；职业操守

falsification [ˌfɔːlsɪfɪ'keɪʃn] *n.* 伪造；歪曲

fraud [frɔːd] *n.* 欺诈，骗局，诡计

commitment [kə'mɪtmənt] *n.* 奉献，投入；热情，决心；义务，责任

adequately ['ædɪkwətli] *adv.* 充分地，足够地；适当地

competent ['kɑːmpɪtənt] *adj.* 能干的，能胜任的

authorize ['ɔːθəraɪz] *v.* 批准，许可；授权

validate ['vælɪdeɪt] *v.* 批准，确认……有效

intermediate [ˌɪntər'miːdiət] *n.* （化合物）中间体

Notes

Pharmaceutical Administration Law of the People's Republic of China 中华人民共和国药品管理法

Regulations for Implementation of the Pharmaceutical Administration Law of the People's Republic of China 中华人民共和国药品管理实施条例

Translation

药品生产质量管理规范

第一章 总则

第一条 为规范药品生产质量管理，根据《中华人民共和国药品管理法》《中华人民共和国药品管理法实施条例》，制定本规范。

第二条 企业应当建立药品质量管理体系。该体系应当涵盖影响药品质量的所有因素，包括确保药品质量符合预定用途的有组织、有计划的全部活动。

第三条 本规范作为质量管理体系的一部分，是药品生产管理和质量控制的基本要求，旨在最大限度地降低药品生产过程中污染、交叉污染以及混淆、差错等风险，确保持续稳定地生产出符合预定用途和注册要求的药品。

第四条 企业应当严格执行本规范，坚持诚实守信，禁止任何虚假、欺骗行为。

第二章 质量管理

第一节 原则

第五条 企业应当建立符合药品质量管理要求的质量目标，将药品注册的有关安全、有效和质量可控的所有要求，系统地贯彻到药品生产、控制及产品放行、贮存、发运的全过程中，确保所生产的药品符合预定用途和注册要求。

第六条 企业高层管理人员应当确保实现既定的质量目标，不同层次的人员以及供应商、经销商应当共同参与并承担各自的责任。

第七条 企业应当配备足够的、符合要求的人员、厂房、设施和设备，为实现质量目标提供必要的条件。

第三节 质量控制

第十一条 质量控制包括相应的组织机构、文件系统以及取样、检验等，确保物料或产品在放行前完成必要的检验，确认其质量符合要求。

第十二条 质量控制的基本要求

（1）应当配备适当的设施、设备、仪器和经过培训的人员，有效、可靠地完成所有质量控制的相关活动。

（2）应当有批准的操作规程，用于原辅料、包装材料、中间产品、待包装产品和成品的取样、检查、检验以及产品的稳定性考察，必要时进行环境监测，以确保符合本规范的要求。

（3）由经授权的人员按照规定的方法对原辅料、包装材料、中间产品、待包装产品和成品取样。

（4）检验方法应当经过验证或确认。

（5）取样、检查、检验应当有记录，偏差应当经过调查并记录。

（6）物料、中间产品、待包装产品和成品必须按照质量标准进行检查和检验，并有记录。

……

Unit 5   Pharmaceutical Operation

Lead-in

Drugs cannot be directly administrated to patients. Before clinical use, they must be transformed into proper forms according to the application route, packaging and approval. The physical state of drugs along with the other components comprise the dosage forms. Common dosage forms include tablets, injections, capsules, sterile powders for injection, ointments and suppositories. Pharmaceutical manufacturing is the process of industrial-scale, commercial preparation of a drug product according to clinical requirements.

In-depth Reading

Preview questions

1. What are the advantages of tablets?
2. What are the five main categories of excipients?

Text

The Preparation of Tablets

Tablets are solid dosage forms, which contain drugs and suitable excipients in the shape of round or special-shaped solid preparations. Partly due to the bulky volume of highly dispersed powders or granules, which makes storage and transportation less convenient, compression into tablets is highly desirable.

Advantages of tablets include: accurate dosing; very good physicochemical properties;

convenience in transportation and administration; low manufacturing cost; versatility to accommodate different clinical requirements, for instance oral disintegrating tablets for fast release, sustained-release tablets for long duration of action, buccal tablets for local action in the mouth and vaginal tablets for topical use within the vagina.

Disadvantages of tablets include inconvenience for swallowing by infants, children and the elderly, complexity in formulation and production, and stringent requirements for quality control.

Excipients are all materials in a tablet formulation that are not the drug. Besides providing the needed function, excipients in a tablet should be highly stable, unreactive with the active ingredients, non-toxic, non-hazardous and devoid of adverse effects. Excipients can be classified into five main categories based on the function:

(1) Diluents   Diluents are also called as fillers. It is commonly acceptable that tablets with diameters less than 6mm or mass less than 100mg are not convenient for administration. The purpose of diluents in tablets is to increase the mass or volume of the tablets. More importantly, diluents are chosen to improve the compressibility of drug powders and ensure content uniformity, especially for tablets of low doses.

(2) Moistening agents and binders   Moistening agents and binders are excipients added during granulation to facilitate aggregation of powders.

(3) Disintegrants   Disintegrants refer to excipients that drive tablets to disassemble into fine particles in the gastrointestinal tract.

(4) Lubricants   Lubricants is a broad concept, and there are three types of excipients that act as lubricants: glidants, anti-adherents and lubricants.

(5) Conditioning agent for color, flavor and taste   The flavor, taste and appearance are modified by the addition of conditioning agents.

Examples

(1) Compound sulfamethoxazole tablets
[Formulation]

Sulfamethoxazole (SMZ)	400g
Trimethoprim (TMP)	80g
Starch	40g

10% Starch paste	24g
Dry starch	23g(4%)
Magnesium stearate	3g(0.5%)
Yield 1000 tablets	0. 4g SMZ/tablet

〔Preparation〕

Screen SMZ and TMP with an 80-mesh (1mesh=0.254mm) sieve; mix with starch; add starch paste to make soft materials; extrude through a 14-mesh sieve to make wet granules; dry at 70-80℃ ; screen with a 12-mesh sieve; add dry starch and magnesium stearate ; mix homogeneously and compress into tablets.

(2) Compound acetylsalicylic acid tablets (aspirin tablets)

〔Formulation〕

Aspirin	268g
Acetaminophen	136g
Caffeine	33.4g
Starch	266g
Starch paste (15% - 17%)	85g
Talc (5%)	25g
Light liquid paraffin	2.5g
Tartaric acid	2.7g
Yield 1000 tablets	0.268g aspirin/tablet

〔Preparation〕

Mix caffeine, acetaminophen and 1/3 starch homogenously; add starch paste to make soft material; extrude through a 14-mesh nylon sieve to make wet granules; dry at 70℃ ; screen with a 12-mesh nylon sieve; add the other 2/3 starch(pre-dried at 100-105℃)and talc adsorbed with liquid paraffin; mix and screen with 12-mesh sieve ; compress into 12 mm tablets.

Vocabulary

clinical〔'klɪnɪkl〕*adj.* 临床的

transform [træns'fɔːrm] v. 使改观，使变形，使转化

route [ruːt] n. 路线，航线；道路，路途；途径，方法

comprise [kəm'praɪz] v. 包括，包含；构成，组成

tablet ['tæblət] n. 药片，片剂

injection [ɪn'dʒekʃn] n. 注射剂

capsule ['kæpsl] n. 胶囊

sterile powder 无菌粉

ointment ['ɔɪntmənt] n. 药膏

dosage form 剂型

excipient [ɪk'sɪpɪənt] n. 辅料

bulky ['bʌlki] adj. 笨重的，庞大的

volume ['vɑːljəm] n. 体积，容积；（成套图书中的）卷，册

dispersed [dɪ'spɜːrst] adj. 散布的；被分散的

granule ['grænjuːl] n. 颗粒剂

dosing ['dosɪŋ] n. 定量给料，配量

transportation [ˌtrænspər'teɪʃn] n. 运输，运送

versatility [ˌvɜːrsə'tɪləti] n. 多功能性；多才多艺；用途广泛

oral disintegrating tablet 口腔崩解片

stringent ['strɪndʒənt] adj. 严格的

diluent ['dɪljʊənt] n. 稀释剂

compressibility [kəmˌpresɪ'bɪlɪti] n. 压缩性

moistening agent 润湿剂

disintegrant [dɪs'ɪntəgrənt] n. 分解质，崩解剂

gastrointestinal [ˌgæstrovɪn'testɪnl] adj. 胃肠的

lubricant ['luːbrɪkənt] n. 润滑剂

glidant ['glaɪdənt] n. 助滑剂，助流剂

antiadherent 抗黏剂

flavor ['fleɪvər] n. 风味

appearance [ə'pɪrəns] n. 外表，外观

trimethoprim [traɪ'meθəprɪm] n. 甲氧苄氨嘧啶，甲氧苄啶

starch [stɑːrtʃ] n. 淀粉

magnesium stearate 硬脂酸镁

yield [jiːld] v. 产生（收益、效益等）；出产（天然产品、工业产品）

mesh [meʃ] *n.* 网，网状物；目数

80-mesh sieve 80 目筛

extrude [ɪk ˈstruːd] *v.* 挤出，压出

homogeneously [ˌhoməˈdʒinɪrslɪ] *adv.* 同样地，同类地

aspirin [ˈæsprɪn] *n.* 阿司匹林

acetaminophen [əˌsiːtəˈmɪnəfen] *n.* 对乙酰氨基酚

talc [tælk] *n.* 滑石粉，爽身粉

paraffin [ˈpærəfɪn] *n.* 石蜡

tartaric acid 酒石酸

nylon [ˈnaɪlɑːn] *n.* 尼龙

Notes

compound sulfamethoxazole tablet：复方磺胺甲噁唑片（复方新诺明片）

Translation

片剂的制备

片剂指原料药物与适宜的辅料制成的圆形的或异形的片状固体制剂。由于呈分散状态的散剂、颗粒剂体积大，在贮存、运输、使用过程中多有不便，于是考虑将其压制成片状，以缩小体积，方便使用。

片剂的优点包括：剂量准确；物理化学性能较好；运输携带方便；生产成本低；可以满足不同临床医疗的需要，如速效片、缓释片、口腔局部用药（口含片）、阴道局部用药（阴道片）等。

片剂的缺点是婴幼儿、老年患者不易吞服，并且处方与制备工艺较为复杂，质量控制要求高。

辅料指片剂处方中除药物以外所有附加物的总称。片剂辅料除具备其本身应有的功能外，还应具备良好的物理化学稳定性，不与主药发生任何物理化学反应；对人体无毒、无害、无不良反应。根据各种辅料所起的作用不同，将辅料分为五大类：

（1）稀释剂　稀释剂亦称作填充剂。片剂的直径一般不小于 6mm，质量多在 100mg 以上，否则不便使用。稀释剂的作用不仅是增加片剂的质量（或体积），更重要的是改善药物的压缩成形性，提高含量均匀度，特别是小剂量药物的片剂。

（2）润湿剂和黏合剂　润湿剂和黏合剂是在制粒时添加的物料，以使物料黏结，

方便制粒。

（3）崩解剂　崩解剂是促使片剂在胃肠液中碎裂成细小颗粒的辅料。

（4）润滑剂　润滑剂是一个广义的概念，是助流剂、抗黏剂、润滑剂的总称。

（5）色、香、味调节剂　为了改善口味和外观，经常在片剂中加入着色剂、芳香剂和甜味剂等。

片剂实例

例1：复方磺胺甲噁唑片

[配方]

磺胺甲噁唑 (SMZ)	400g
甲氧苄啶 (TMP)	80g
淀粉	40g
10% 淀粉浆	24g
干淀粉	23g (4% 左右)
硬脂酸镁	3g (0.5% 左右)
制成 1000 片	每片含 SMZ 0.4g

[制备]

将 SMZ 和 TMP 分别过 80 目筛，与淀粉混匀，加淀粉浆制软材，用 14 目筛挤出制湿颗粒，于 70～80℃干燥，用 12 目筛整粒，加入干淀粉及硬脂酸镁混匀后压片，即得。

例2：复方阿司匹林（乙酰水杨酸）片

[配方]

阿司匹林	268g
对乙酰氨基酚（扑热息痛）	136g
咖啡因	33.4g
淀粉	266g
淀粉浆 (15%~ 17%)	85g
滑石粉 (5%)	25g
轻质液状石蜡	2.5g
酒石酸	2.7g
制成 1000 片	每片含阿司匹林 0.268g

［制备］

将咖啡因、对乙酰氨基酚与淀粉总量的 1/3 混匀，加酒石酸、淀粉浆制软材，过 14 目尼龙筛制得颗粒，于 70℃干燥，干颗粒用 12 目尼龙筛整粒，最后加剩余 2/3 的淀粉（预先在 100～105℃干燥）及吸附有液状石蜡的滑石粉共同混匀后再过 12 目尼龙筛，冲压成 12mm 片剂，即得。

Quiz

Ⅰ. Answer the questions according to the text.

1. What do the common dosage forms include?

_____

2. What are the disadvantages of tablets?

_____

3. Why diluents is necessary in tablets?

_____

4. What are the roles of disintegrants?

_____

Ⅱ. Complete the sentences with the words given. Change the form if necessary.

| capsule | stringent | gastrointestinal | yield |
| clinical | transportation | flavor | appearance |

1. He announced that there would be more _____ controls on the possession of weapons.

2. The patient swallowed the _____ without drinking water.

3. This year's _____ of wheat is higher than ever before.

4. She had always prided herself on her _____ .

5. The new museum must be accessible by public _____ .

6. Rice cake can be made into original _____ or various other flavors.

7. The new drug is undergoing _____ trials.

8. Beans and legumes are rich in fiber, which is good for _____ health and may help prevent colon cancer.

Ⅲ. Translation between English and Chinese.

pharmaceutical operation	生产成本低
dosage form	80 目筛
solid dosage form	制软材
convenience in transportation and administration	制湿颗粒
tablet with diameter less than 6mm	非药用部分

Extended Reading

Text

Preparation of Granules

Granules are dry particulate preparations of a definite particle size, comprised of APIs (active pharmaceutical ingredients) and suitable excipients. Granules are primarily designed for oral administration, either by direct swallowing or after dispersing into water. There are several categories of granules, including soluble granules, suspending granules, effervescent granules, enteric granules, sustained-release granules and controlled-release granules.

The flow chart of the preparation of granules is shown in Fig. 5-1. Granulation is one of the key techniques frequently used in production of granules, capsules and tablets. The aim of granulation is to prevent dust generation, improve and enhance compressibility and filling properties. Based on whether a wetting agent or a binder is used or not, granulation can be classified into wet granulation and dry granulation.

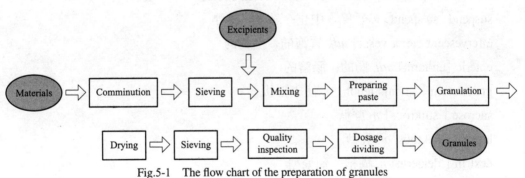

Fig.5-1　The flow chart of the preparation of granules

Excipients commonly used in granules include diluents and binders, as well as disintegrants, if needed. Frequently used diluents for granules include starch, sucrose, lactose, and dextrin. Starch paste and cellulose derivatives are the most commonly used binders.

Procedures for preparation of granules are as follows.

(1) Kneading　Kneading is a key process in wet granulation. The mixture of the drugs and suitable excipients is blended first and kneaded after addition of binders to obtain wet

materials.

(2) Granulation   Conventional extrusion method is commonly employed to produce wet granules. In recent years, modern granulation techniques, such as fluid-bed granulation and blending granulation, have been used as well.

(3) Drying   The wet granules produced should be dried immediately to avoid agglomeration and compression-induced deformation in common ovens or fluid-bed dryers. In an oven dryer, the wet materials stay static, which is favorable for keeping the size and shape of the granules. However, the granules are prone to agglomerate and therefore they need manual, intermittent stirring. In a fluid-bed dryer where the wet granules are dried dynamically—a process that might crush the granules but limit agglomeration.

(4) Screening and sieving   Dried granules are screened and sieved in order to disperse agglomerated granules, on the other hand, obtain granules of uniform size.

(5) Quality control and dosage dividing   The sieved granules are sealed in suitable package bags after subjecting to analysis of drug content and particle size measurement.

Vocabulary

API (active pharmaceutical ingredient) 活性药物成分

suspend [sə'spend] v. 暂停，中止；悬浮，漂浮

effervescent [ˌefər'vesnt] adj. 冒泡的，沸腾的

enteric [en'terɪk] adj. 肠的；肠溶的

granulation [ˌɡrænjə'leɪʃən] n. 使成粒状

sucrose ['suːkroʊs] n. 蔗糖

lactose ['læktoʊs] n. 乳糖

dextrin ['dekstrɪn] n. 糊精；葡聚糖

cellulose ['seljuloʊs] n. 纤维素

derivative [dɪ'rɪvətɪv] n. 衍生物

kneading ['niːdɪŋ] n. 捏合

granulation technique 制粒技术

fluid-bed granulation 流化床制粒

blending granulation 搅拌制粒

agglomeration [əˌɡlɑːmə'reɪʃn] n. 凝聚，结块

compression [kəm'preʃn] n. 压紧，压缩

deformation [ˌdiːfɔːrˈmeɪʃn] *n.* 变形

compression-induced deformation 受挤压变形

static [ˈstætɪk] *adj.* 静止的，停滞的

intermittent [ˌɪntərˈmɪtənt] *adj.* 间歇的，断断续续的

stir [stɜːr] *v.* 搅拌，搅和

dynamically [daɪˈnæmɪkli] *adv.* 动态地；充满活力地；不断变化地

screen [skriːn] *v.* 筛，筛选

seal in 封入

flowability [flaʊəˈbɪlɪti] *n.* 流动性

Translation

颗粒剂的制备

颗粒剂指原料药物与适宜的辅料混合制成的具有一定粒度的干燥颗粒状制剂。颗粒剂主要用于口服，可直接吞服或冲入水中饮服。颗粒剂可分为可溶颗粒、混悬颗粒、泡腾颗粒、肠溶颗粒、缓释颗粒和控释颗粒。

颗粒剂的制备工艺流程如图 5-1 所示。在颗粒剂、胶囊剂与片剂生产中，制粒技术是关键技术之一，且有广泛运用。通过制粒，可以减少粉尘飞扬，改善压缩性与填充性。根据润湿剂或黏合剂使用与否，将制粒方法分为湿法制粒与干法制粒。

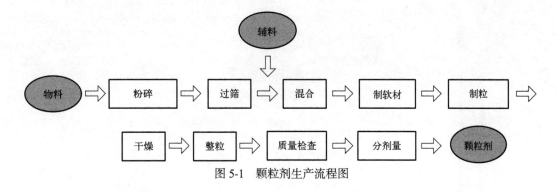

图 5-1　颗粒剂生产流程图

颗粒剂中常用的辅料有稀释剂、黏合剂，有时根据需要也可加入崩解剂。颗粒剂中常用的稀释剂有淀粉、蔗糖、乳糖、糊精等。常用的黏合剂有淀粉浆、纤维素衍生物等。

制备颗粒的具体操作步骤如下：

(1) 制软材　制软材是湿法制粒的关键技术。将药物与适宜的辅料混合均匀后，加入适当的黏合剂，即制得软材。

(2) 制粒　通常采用传统的挤出制粒法制备湿颗粒。近年来流化床制粒、搅拌制粒等现代制粒技术也应用于颗粒剂的制备中。

(3) 干燥　制得的湿颗粒应立即进行干燥，以防止结块或受压变形。常用的干燥方法有箱式干燥法、流化床干燥法。箱式干燥法使物料静态干燥，颗粒的大小和形状不易变，但颗粒间容易粘连，需要人工方法进行间歇搅动；流化床干燥法使物料动态干燥，颗粒易碎，但不易粘连。

(4) 整粒与分级　将干燥后的颗粒通过筛分法进行整粒和分级，一方面使结块、粘连的颗粒散开，另一方面可获得均匀的颗粒。

(5) 质量检查与分剂量　将制得的颗粒进行含量检查与粒度测定等，按剂量装入包装袋中。

Unit 6　Traditional Chinese Medicine Processing

Lead-in

Processing of Chinese medicinals is the techniques to deal with Chinese medicinals based on traditional Chinese medicinal theories and according to the nature of medicinals and different requirements in forms of prescription, preparation and therapy. The purpose of processing Chinese medicinals can be summarized as follows:

(1) To reduce or eliminate the toxicity and side effects to guarantee medication safety;

(2) To enhance medicinal actions and increase therapeutic effects;

(3) To modify the natures and efficacy of medicinals to meet the requirements of patients' conditions;

(4) To change the properties and forms to make it easier for storage and preparation;

(5) To purify medicinal materials to guarantee their quality and accurate mass;

(6) To get rid of unpleasant smells to make it easier for taking.

In-depth Reading

Preview questions

1. List the five categories of processing Chinese medicinals.

2. Stir-frying can be subdivided into 3 categories, what are they?

Text

Methods of Processing Chinese Medicinals

The methods of processing Chinese medicinals are various. Generally speaking, they fall into the following five categories.

1. Purifying and cutting

It consists of three working procedures: purifying, grinding and cutting.

(1) Purifying   Purifying is the method of taking away the earth, impurities and non-pharmaceutical parts to make the medicinals clean and pure by selecting, sieving, winnowing, brushing, scraping, digging or striking, such as picking out the branches and leaves of Xinyi (辛夷), winnowing the impurities in Yiyiren (薏苡仁), brushing away the villus on the back of Pipaye (枇杷叶), scarping away the coarse bark of Rougui (肉桂), and striking away the solid spine of Baijili (白蒺藜).

(2) Grinding   Grinding is the method of grinding medicinal materials into pieces by pounding, grinding, or filing to make it easier for further processing, preparation and taking orally, such as the pounding of Muli (牡蛎), the grinding of Chuanbeimu (川贝母), and the filing of horn medicinals.

(3) Cutting   Medicinal drugs can be cut into slices, segments, sections or shreds for the convenience in further processing, preparation and storage. Cutting the medicinals into small pieces may be helpful to acquire the active ingredients when decocted and thus improve the quality of decoction. For instance, Tianma (天麻) should be cut into thin slices, Zexie (泽泻) into thick slices, Huangqi (黄芪) into oblique slices, Gancao (甘草) into round slices.

2. Processing with water

Processing with water is the method of processing medicinal materials with clean water of lower temperature and other liquid adjuvants. The specific methods are rinsing and washing, soaking, moistening, spraying and powder-refining with water. The main purposes are to clean and soften them, to remove the impurities, to cut them easily, to lower toxicity, or to adjust medicinal properties. For instance, Lugen (芦根) should be washed off the dirt and impurities, Haizao (海藻) should be rinsed the salinity, Fuzi (附子) should be soaked with brine.

3. Processing with fire

Processing with fire is the method of processing medicinal materials by heating with fire, with purpose of changing medicinal properties, improving medicinal effects, reducing or lowering medicinal toxicity, and making the medicinal crisp and convenient for later preparations and administration. The common methods are stir- frying, calcining and roasting.

(1) Stir-frying   Stir-frying is the method of putting medicinal materials in a pan to heat and stir them repeatedly till the required degree. It is divided into plain frying and frying with adjuvants. Plain frying is putting medicinal materials in a pan to heat and stir without adding any adjuvants. It is subdivided into "frying to yellow（炒黄）" "frying to brown（炒焦）" "frying to charcoal（炒炭）". The typical medicinals are fried Niubangzi（牛蒡子）, burnt Shanzha（山楂）and Aiye（艾叶）charcoal.

(2) Calcining   Calcining is the method of heating and frying medicinals directly or indirectly with strong fire. It can be classified into directly calcining（明煅）and covered calcining（焖煅）. The former refers to putting solid mineral or oracle bone on strong fire to calcine directly, such as Duanmuli（煅牡蛎）and Duanshigao（煅石膏）. Covered calcining refers to putting medicinal material in covered container while heating, such as Xueyutan（血余炭）and Zonglütan（棕榈炭）.

(3) Roasting   Roasting is the method of wrapping medicinal materials with wet flour or wet paper and then heating them in hot ashes or heating after putting them on different layers of straw paper , such as roasting Gegen（葛根）and Muxiang（木香）.

4. Processing with both water and fire

This method of processing medicinal materials involves both water and fire, and sometimes other adjuvants. The purposes are to change medicinal properties, to improve therapeutic effects, and to reduce or eliminate toxicity or side effects. The common methods include boiling, roasting, steaming, quenching and blanching.

5. Other processing methods

Besides the above-mentioned four, there are other special processing methods, such as crystallizing, sprouting and fermenting.

Vocabulary

medicinal [mə'dɪsɪnl] *adj.* 药用的，有疗效的；*n.* 药用物质，药用材料

theory ['θiːəri] *n.* 学说，理论

prescription [prɪ'skrɪpʃn] *n.* 处方，药方；处方药；开处方，开药方

preparation [ˌprepə'reɪʃn] *n.* 准备；制剂

therapy ['θerəpi] *n.* 治疗，疗法

toxicity [tɑːk 'sɪsəti] *n.* 毒性

guarantee [ˌgærən'tiː] *v.* 确保，保证

storage [ˈstɔːrɪdʒ] n. 贮存，贮藏

accurate [ˈækjərət] adj. 准确的，精确的

purify [ˈpjʊrɪfaɪ] v. 使（某物）洁净，净化

procedure [prəˈsiːdʒər] n. 手续，步骤；程序；外科手术；应用程序

grind [graɪnd] v. 磨碎，碾碎；使锋利

sieve [sɪv] n. 筛子；滤网；v. 筛；滤

strike [straɪk] v. 打，撞；（用手或武器等）打

villus [ˈvɪləs] n. 绒毛；长茸毛

coarse [kɔːrs] adj. 粗糙的，粗织的；粗的，大颗粒的；粗鲁的

spine [spaɪn] n. 刺

pound [paʊnd] v. 连续重击，猛打

file [faɪl] v. 归档，存档；锉

horn [hɔːrn] n. 角；角质

shred [ʃred] n. 细条，碎片

ingredient [ɪnˈɡriːdiənt] n. 成分，原料

decoct [diˈkɑːkt] v. 煎；熬

adjuvant [ˈædʒəvənt] adj. 辅助的；n. 佐药；辅助物

rinse [rɪns] v. （用清水）冲洗

moisten [ˈmɔɪsn] v. 弄湿；使……湿润；变潮湿

stir-frying 炒

calcine [ˈkælsaɪn] v. 煅烧，焙烧；（使）氧化；n. 煅烧产物

roast [roʊst] v. 炙，烘

plain frying 清炒

charcoal [ˈtʃɑːrkoʊl] n. 木炭

straw paper 草浆纸，草纸

crystallize [ˈkrɪstəlaɪz] v. （使）结晶

sprout [spraʊt] v. （植物）发芽，抽条；n. 苗，新芽，嫩枝

ferment [fərˈment] v. （使）发酵

Notes

powder-refining with water 水飞法。利用粗细粉末在水中悬浮性不同，将不溶于水的药材与水共研，经反复研磨制备成极细腻粉末的方法。水飞法适用于不溶于水的矿物药（如朱砂、雄黄、炉甘石）及贝壳类中药。

Translation

中药的炮制方法

中药的炮制方法多种多样，总的说来，可分为以下5类。

1. 修治

包括3种工序：净化、粉碎和切制。

（1）净化（纯净药材）　通过挑拣、筛、簸、刷、刮、挖、撞等方法，除去药材中的泥土、杂质和非药用部分，使药材纯净。如拣去辛夷的枝、叶，簸去薏苡仁的杂质，刷除枇杷叶背面的绒毛，刮去肉桂的粗皮，撞去白蒺藜的硬刺等。

（2）粉碎（药材）　通过捣、磨、锉等方法，使药材达到一定粉碎度，便于调配、制剂或服用。如牡蛎的捣碎、川贝母的研粉、角类药的锉粉等。

（3）切制（药材）　将药材切为片、段、丝、块等，便于调配、制剂或贮存。切制利于有效成分煎出，提高煎药质量。如天麻切薄片，泽泻切厚片，黄芪切斜片，甘草切圆片等。

2. 水制

水制是以较低温度的清水或其他液体辅料处理药材的方法。常用的方法有漂洗、浸泡、闷润、喷洒、水飞等。其主要目的是清洁药物、除去杂质、软化药物、便于切制、降低毒性及调整药性等。如芦根洗去泥土等杂质，海藻漂去盐分，胆巴水浸泡附子等。

3. 火制

火制是将药物用火加热，以改变其药性，增加药效，降低毒性，便于制剂和服用。常见方式有炒、煅、煨。

（1）炒　是指将药物置锅中加热，不断翻动，炒至一定"火候"即可。炒法分为清炒和加辅料炒两类。清炒是将药物放置锅内，不加辅料直接翻炒。清炒又有炒黄、炒焦和炒炭之分。如炒牛蒡子、焦山楂、艾叶炭等。

（2）煅　用猛火直接或间接煅烧药材的方法。可分为明煅和焖煅。前者是指将坚硬的矿物或甲骨类药材直接煅烧，如煅牡蛎、煅石膏等。焖煅指将药物密闭煅烧，如血余炭、棕榈炭。

（3）煨　将药材用湿面粉或湿纸包裹置于火灰中，或用草纸与药物隔层分开加热的方法。如煨葛根、煨木香等。

4. 水火共制

这类炮制方法既要用水又要用火，有些药物还必须加入其他辅料进行炮制。其目的是改变药物性能，增强药效，降低或消除药物的毒性和副作用。常用的方法有煮、炙、蒸、淬、燀等。

5. 其他制法

除上述4种方法外，还有其他制法，例如制霜、发芽、发酵法。

Quiz

I. Answer the questions according to the text.

1. What are the purposes of processing Chinese medicinals?

_____

2. What procedures do purifying and cutting consist of?

_____

3. Which method is Chuanbeimu（川贝母）suited to?

_____

4. What are the differences between directly calcining and covered calcining?

_____

II. Complete the sentences with the words given. Change the form if necessary.

| prescription | preparation | storage | sieve |
| coarse | accurate | toxicity | therapy |

1. Most leukaemia patients undergo some sort of drug _____.

2. I've been spending a lot more time editing photos, posting online and clearing _____ on my phone.

3. Every chemical has _____ , but it's all in the dose.

4. As a matter of fact, the couple are cleaning their house in _____ for the new baby's coming.

5. An _____ diagnosis was made after a series of tests.

6. Many flu medications are available without a _____ .

7. It's good to have _____ grain often.

8. Press the raspberries through a fine _____ to form a puree.

III. Translation between English and Chinese.

powder-refining with water	水制
stir-frying	火制
straw paper	水火共制
Chinese medicinals	非药用部分
side effect	

Extended Reading

Text

What Is TCM?

The origin of traditional Chinese medicine (TCM) can be traced to Shennongshi, a mythological figure from about 5,000 years ago, who sampled hundreds of herbs for use as medicines. The formal history of TCM started about 2,500 years ago with the Inner Canon of Yellow Emperor, the first written account of his practice. Central to the treatment are the TCM theories of the Yin and Yang, considering the two opposing forces of the body. The Yin represents the cold and passive parts, while the Yang represents the hot and active ones. TCM practitioners believe that when these two parts are out of balance, the smooth flow of qi and blood through paths in the body is disrupted. TCM views a patient's condition as a reflection of the interaction of five elements of nature: wood, fire, earth, metal and water. Each of the elements inter-generates, inter-restricts and inter-transforms the other and achieves a balance. The goal is to treat each patient holistically, with prescriptions tailored to the individual patient's condition.

Chinese people generally perceive TCM as more effective for disease and chronic illness prevention, and they view western medicine as being more effective for acute and serious illnesses. Another major difference between TCM and western medicine is that, until recently, TCM has relied on patient experience, not clinical trials, for proof of effectiveness.

TCM combines raw materials, principally herbs, to treat disease. Historically, the formulation incorporated as many as 10,000 ingredients, 90 percent extracted from herbs and 10 percent from animal and minerals. Today, practitioners of TCM regularly use around 300 ingredients in their widely available formulations.

The principle used for combining ingredients has its origins in the framework of Monarch-Minister-Assistant-Guide, which was documented 5,000 years ago in the Shennong's Classic of Materia Medica. The framework includes a chief herb, or main ingredient of a formula; the ministerial herb, ancillary to the imperial herb, which augments and promotes the action of the main ingredient; the assistant herb, which reduces side effects of the imperial herb; and the servant herb, which harmonizes or coordinates the actions of the other herbs.

Traditional Chinese Medicine has made great contribution to the health of Chinese people, and it became an independent medical system in world medical field with its special clinical effect, rational theory system and rich practice experience. Chinese government has put great importance to Traditional Chinese Medicine, formulating a series of guiding principles and policies to support and promote TCM development. TCM is now on its way to become a widely accepted healing approach worldwide.

Vocabulary

Traditional Chinese Medicine 中医

mythological [ˌmɪθəˈlɑːdʒɪkl] *adj.* 神话的；神话学的；虚构的

herb [ɜːrb] *n.* 药草，香草；草本植物

Inner Canon of Yellow Emperor 黄帝内经

practitioner [prækˈtɪʃənər] *n.* 从业人员，执业者

holistically [hoʊˈlɪstɪkli] *adv.* 整体地；全盘地

tailor [ˈteɪlər] *n.* 裁缝；*v.* 定做（衣服）；迎合，使适应

chronic [ˈkrɑːnɪk] *adj.* （疾病）慢性的，长期的

raw [rɔː] *adj.* 生的，未煮过的；天然的，未经加工的

byproduct [ˈbaɪˌprɑːdʌkt] *n.* 副产品

framework [ˈfreɪmwɜːrk] *n.* 构架，结构；参照标准，准则

Shennong's Classic of Materia Medica 神农本草经

ancillary [ˈænsəleri] *adj.* 辅助的；副的；从属的；*n.* 助手；附件

augment [ɔːɡˈment] *v.* 增加，增大；加强，补充

harmonize [ˈhɑːrmənaɪz] *v.* 使和谐；使一致

Notes

Monarch-Minister-Assistant-Guide 君臣佐使　中医配制药方的方法。用于主治的称君，辅治或治兼证的称臣，相反而相助的称佐，引导及调和的称使。

Translation

中医

传统中医的起源可以追溯到神农氏，一个大约 5000 年前的神话人物，他采集了数百种草药作为药物。中医有文字记录的历史始于大约 2500 年前的《黄帝内经》，这

是中医实践的第一部书籍。中医治疗的核心是阴阳理论，阴阳被认为是身体的两种对立力量。阴代表寒冷、抑制的部分，而阳代表温热和主动的部分。中医师认为，当这两个部分失去平衡时，人体气脉将不能顺畅流动。中医认为病人的病情反映了木、火、土、金和水五种自然元素的相互作用：每个元素相生、相克，实现平衡。中医的理念是对每位患者进行整体治疗，并根据患者的具体情况开处方。中国人普遍认为中医药对疾病的预防和慢性病的治疗更有效，西药对急性和严重疾病更有效。中医和西医之间的另一个主要区别是，中医一直依靠诊治经验而不是临床试验来证明疗效。

中医用中药配伍进行治疗，其中主要是草药。发展至今，中药种类多达 10000 种，90% 为草药，10% 为动物和矿物药。如今，中医师广泛使用的配方大约有 300 种。

中药配伍原则源于"君臣佐使"，这一原则在 5000 多年以前的《神农本草经》上就有记载。该原则中有君药，即配方的主药或主要成分；臣药，附属于君药，增强和促进主要成分的作用；佐药，减少君药的副作用；使药，协调其他几味药的功效。

中医以其独特的临床疗效、合理的理论体系和丰富的实践经验，为中国人民的健康做出了巨大贡献，成为世界医学领域一个独立的医疗体系。我国政府高度重视中医药，制定了一系列支持和促进中医药发展的指导方针和政策。中医药正在成为全世界广泛接受的治疗方法。

Unit 7   Drugs Quality Control

Lead-in

The pharmacopoeia is a code, which contains the standards and specifications for the drugs in a country. It describes the official title (generic or non-proprietary name) , source, physical properties identification, purity test, content (potency, or activity) determination, classification, dosage, specification, storage, preparation of listed drugs.

In-depth Reading

Preview questions

1. What is the requirement about weight variation of tablets?
2. What is the requirement about effervescence volume of tablets?

Text

Tablets Quality Control

According to the Chinese Pharmacopoeia, unless otherwise specified, tablets should comply with the following requirements.

1. Weight variation

Tablets should comply with the following requirements.

Weigh accurately 20 tablets and calculate the average weight; then weigh individually each of the 20 tablets and compare the weight of each tablets with the average weight (if assay is not required, the weight of each tablet should be compared with the labelled weight) . Not more than 2 of the individual weights shall deviate from the average weight by more than the weight variation limit shown in Table 7-1, and none deviate by more than twice the limit.

Before being coated with sugar , the tablet cores should comply with the test for weight variation. Sugar coated tablets are not required to comply with the test for weight variation while film coated tablets are required to comply with it. Where the test for content uniformity is specified, the test for weight variation may not be required.

Table 7-1   Weight variation requirements for tablets

Average weight of labelled weight	Weight variation limit
Less than 0.30g	$\pm 7.5\%$
Not less than 0.30g	$\pm 5.0\%$

2. Disintegration

Unless otherwise specified, tablets should comply with the determination of disintegration. Vaginal tablets should comply with the disintegration test for suppositories and vaginal tablets. Chewable tablets may not be required to comply with the test for disintegration. Where dissolution test or drug release test is specified, disintegration test may not be required.

3. Effervescence volume

Effervescent vaginal tablets should comply with the following requirements.

Add 2mL or 4mL of water (according to Table7-2 below) , accurately measured, to ten 25mL graduated test tubes with stoppers (the internal diameter is 1.5cm; if the tablet is large, the internal diameter is 2.0cm) separately, place them in a water bath at 37℃ ±1℃ for 5 minutes. Add 1 tablet to each of the ten test tubes, stopper the test tubes for 20 minutes, and examine the maximum volume of effervescence. The average volume of effervescence should not be less than 6 mL, and not more than 2 tablets should be in average effervescence volumes of less than 4 mL.

Table 7-2   Effervescence volume requirements

Average weight	Added water/mL
Less than 1.5g	2.0
Not less than 1.5g	4.0

4. Uniformity of dispersion

Dispersible tablets should comply with the following requirements.

The internal diameter of stainless steel sieve is 710μm while the water temperature is 15-25℃. Six tablets should be disintegrated and should pass through the sieve within 3 minutes.

5. Microbial limit

Tablets containing non-monomer active ingredients from animal, plant herb or mineral origin, biological product tablets, tablets for local administration (such as buccal tablets, soluble tablets for external use, vaginal tablets, effervescent vaginal tablets, etc.), should comply with the test for microbial limit of nonsterile products. The results should comply with the requirements.

Vocabulary

generic [dʒə'nerɪk] *adj.* 一般的，通用的

non-proprietary name 非专利药名

variation [ˌveri 'eɪʃn] *n.* 变化，变动

assay [ə'seɪ] *n.* 化验；试验

core [kɔːr] *n.* 果核；中心部分；核心

sugar coated tablet 糖衣片

film coated tablet 薄膜衣片

effervescence [ˌefər'vesns] *n.* 冒泡；泡腾

graduated ['ɡrædʒueɪtɪd] *adj.* 分等级的，分阶段的；标有刻度的

test tube 试管

internal diameter 内直径

water bath 水浴

uniformity of dispersion 分散均匀性

stainless steel 不锈钢

monomer ['mɑːnəmər] *n.* 单体；单元结构

buccal tablet 口含片，口腔贴片

sterile ['sterəl] *adj.* 无菌的

Translation

片剂的质量检查

根据《中华人民共和国药典》，除另有规定外，片剂应进行以下相应检查。

1. 重量差异

照下述方法检查，应符合规定。

取供试品 20 片，求得平均片重后，再分别精密称定每片的重量，每片重量与平均片重比较（凡无含量测定的片剂，每片重量应与标示片重比较），按表 7-1 中的规定，超出重量差异限度的不得多于 2 片，并不得有 1 片超出限度 1 倍。

表 7-1　片剂重量差异要求

平均片重或标示片重	重量差异限度
0.30g 以下	±7.5%
0.30g 及 0.30g 以上	±5.0%

糖衣片的片芯应检查重量差异并符合规定，包糖衣后不再检查重量差异。薄膜衣片应在包薄膜衣后检查重量差异并符合规定。凡规定检查含量均匀度的片剂，一般不再进行重量差异检查。

2. 崩解时限

除另有规定外，片剂照崩解时限检查法检查，应符合规定。阴道片照融变时限检查法检查，应符合规定。咀嚼片不进行崩解时限检查。凡规定检查溶出度、释放度的片剂，一般不再进行崩解时限检查。

3. 发泡量

阴道泡腾片照下述方法检查，应符合规定（表 7-2）。

取 25mL 具塞刻度试管（内径 1.5cm，若片剂直径较大，可改为内径 2.0cm）10 支，按表 7-2 规定分别精密加水 2mL 或 4mL，置（37±1）℃水浴中 5min。各管中分别投入供试品 1 片，塞住试管 20min，观察最大发泡量的体积，平均发泡体积不得少于 6mL，且平均发泡体积少于 4mL 的不得超过 2 片。

表 7-2　发泡体积要求

平均片重	加水量 /mL
1.5g 及 1.5g 以下	2.0
1.5g 以上	4.0

4. 分散均匀性

分散片照下述方法检查，应符合规定。

不锈钢丝网的筛孔内径为 710μm，水温为 15 ～ 25℃；取供试品 6 片，应在 3min 内全部崩解并通过筛网。

5. 微生物限度

以动物、植物、矿物来源的非单体成分制成的片剂，生物制品片剂，以及局部用片剂（如口腔贴片、外用可溶片、阴道片、阴道泡腾片等），照非无菌产品微生物限度检查，结果应符合规定。

Quiz

I. Answer the questions according to the text.

1. If the average weight of the tablets is 0.25g, what should the weight variation limit be ?

_____

2. How many tablets should be used in the weight variation test?

_____

3. Did the film coated tablets need to do the weight variation test?

_____

4. What is the temperature of effervescence volume test ?

_____

II. Complete the sentences with the words given. Change the form if necessary.

assay	sterile	pharmacopoeia	microbial
average	core	variation	individually

1. We need to concentrate on our _____ business.

2. A _____ of a gene can influence people's social behavior.

3. The new edition of the _____ marks a new stage in China's pharmaceutical standards.

4. After chemical _____ , we have known the composition of the ore.

5. _____ injection equipment protects against HBV and HCV transmission.

6. Previously it was thought there were around 100,000 _____ cells in every litre of seawater but scientists now think there could be one billion.

7. These paints can be used _____ or in combination.

8. The _____ of 4, 5 and 9 is 6.

III. Translation between English and Chinese.

water bath	平均重量
not less than 6 mL	糖衣片
stainless steel sieve	内直径
buccal tablet	咀嚼片
vaginal tablet	平均体积

Extended Reading

Text

Capsules

Capsules are solid preparations consisting of drug substances with or without excipients, filled in hollow hard capsules or sealed in soft shells. They may be classified into hard, soft, sustained-release, controlled-release, and enteric-coated capsules. Capsules are mainly intended for oral administration.

(1) Hard capsules (usually known as capsules) Hard capsules are capsules containing a quantity of powders, granules, minitablets, pellets, semisolids or liquids, etc. , with or without suitable excipients, which are produced by suitable preparative technology and enclosed in a hollow capsule shell.

(2) Soft capsules Soft capsules are capsules prepared by enclosing directly a quantity of liquid drug substances, or by enclosing a solution, suspension, emulsion and semisolid, which are made by dissolving or dispersing solid drug substances into soft capsule shells. The soft capsule shells are generally made of gelatin, glycerin or other suitable materials.

(3) Sustained-release capsules Sustained-release capsules are capsules which release drug substances in a gradual, non-constant rate in a specified release medium.

(4) Controlled-release capsules Controlled-release capsules are capsules which release drug substances in a gradual, constant rate in a specified release medium.

(5) Enteric-coated capsules Enteric-coated capsules are hard or soft capsules of which the shell is prepared by suitable enteric-coating material, or are hard capsules filled with granules or pills coated with enteric-coating material. Enteric-coated capsules are insoluble in gastric fluid, but can disintegrate in intestinal fluid to release active ingredients.

Unless otherwise specified, capsules should comply with the following requirements.

(1) Water Water determination for Chinese medicinal hard capsules is required. The water content of the hard capsule is determined by the methods described in determination of water. Unless otherwise specified , the water content is not more than 9.0 percent. Water determination is not required where the contents of hard capsules are liquids or semisolids.

(2) Weight variation Capsules should comply with the following weight variation limit.

Weigh accurately each of 20 capsules (10 capsules for Chinese medicine) , unless otherwise specified. Open each capsule without loss of shell material, and remove the contents as completely as possible: for hard capsules, clean the shell with a small brush; for soft capsules or the hard capsules in which the contents are semisolids or liquids, wash the shell with ether or other volatile solvents, and allow to stand until the odour of the solvents is no longer perceptible. Weigh the shell of each capsule. Calculate the content weight of each capsule and the average weight. Not more than 2 of the individual weights should deviate from the average (or labelled) weight by more than the weight variation limit shown in Table 7-3, and none should deviate by more than twice the limit.

Table 7-3　Weight variation limit for capsules

Average or labelled weight	Weight variation limit
Less than 0.30g	±10%
0.30g or more	±7.5%（±10% for Chinese medicine）

(3) Disintegration test　Unless otherwise specified, capsules, should comply with the determination of disintegration.

(4) Microbial limit　Capsules containing non-monomer active ingredients derived from animal, herb or mineral should comply with the microbiological examination of nonsterile products.

Vocabulary

hollow [ˈhɑːloʊ] adj. 空的，空心的

a quantity of 大量的；一些；许多

enteric-coated 包有肠溶衣的

pellet [ˈpelɪt] n. 芯块，小球

semisolid [ˌsemɪˈsɑːlɪd] adj. 半固体的；n. 半固体

suspension [səˈspenʃn] n. 悬浮液；混悬剂

emulsion [ɪˈmʌlʃn] n. 乳剂

dissolving [dɪˈzɑlvɪŋ] adj. 溶解的；毁灭性的

gelatin [ˈdʒelətɪn] n. 明胶；动物胶；胶制品

odour [ˈoʊdər] n. （尤指难闻的）气味，臭味

ether [ˈiːθər] n. 乙醚

volatile [ˈvɑːlətl] adj. 易挥发的

solvent [ˈsɑːlvənt] n. 溶剂

Notes

sustained-release capsule 缓释胶囊

controlled-release capsule 控释胶囊

enteric-coated capsule 肠溶胶囊

Translation

胶囊剂

胶囊剂系指原料药物或与适宜辅料充填于空心胶囊或密封于软质囊材中制成的固体制剂。胶囊剂可分为硬胶囊、软胶囊、缓释胶囊、控释胶囊、肠溶胶囊等。胶囊主要用于口服。

（1）硬胶囊（通称为胶囊）　系指采用适宜的制剂技术，将原料药物或原料药物加适宜辅料制成的均匀粉末、颗粒、小片、小丸、半固体或液体等，充填于空心胶囊中的胶囊剂。

（2）软胶囊　系指将一定量的液体原料药物直接密封，或将固体原料药物溶解或分散制备成溶液、混悬液、乳状液或半固体，密封于软质囊材中的胶囊剂。软胶囊可用滴制法或压制法制备。软质囊材一般是用明胶、甘油或其他适宜的材料制成。

（3）缓释胶囊　系指在规定的释放介质中缓慢地非恒速释放药物的胶囊剂。

（4）控释胶囊　系指在规定的释放介质中缓慢地恒速释放药物的胶囊剂。

（5）肠溶胶囊　系指用适宜的肠溶材料制备而得的硬胶囊或软胶囊，或用肠溶材料包衣的颗粒或小丸充填于胶囊而制成的硬胶囊。肠溶胶囊不溶于胃液，但能在肠液中崩解而释放活性成分。

除另有规定外，胶囊剂应进行以下相应检查。

（1）水分　中药硬胶囊剂应进行水分检查。取供试品内容物，照水分测定法测定。除另有规定外不得超过9.0%。硬胶囊内容物为液体或半固体者不检查水分。

（2）装量差异　照下述方法检查，应符合规定。

除另有规定外，取供试品20粒（中药取10粒），分别精密称定重量，倾出内容物（不得损失囊壳），硬胶囊囊壳用小刷拭净；软胶囊或内容物为半固体或液体的硬胶囊囊壳用乙醚等易挥发性溶剂洗净，静置直到溶剂挥尽，再分别精密称定囊壳重量，求出每粒内容物的装量与平均装量。每粒装量与平均装量（或标示装量）相比较，超出装量差异限度的不得多于2粒，并不得有1粒超出限度1倍（表7-3）。

表7-3　胶囊剂重量差异限度

平均装量或标示装量	装量差异限度
0.30g以下	±10%
0.30g及0.30g以上	±7.5%（中药±10%）

（3）崩解时限　除另有规定外，照崩解时限检查法检查，均应符合规定。

（4）微生物限度　以动物、植物、矿物质来源的非单体活性成分制成的胶囊剂，生物制品胶囊剂，照非无菌产品微生物限度检查。

Mini Project 2

Section Ⅰ Listening

A patient and a doctor is talking about Traditional Chinese Medicine. Listen carefully, and complete Task 1.

Task 1

1. Mr. Smith used (   ) to cure the patient.

A. acupuncture   B. herb   C. cupping

2. Traditional Chinese Medicine (TCM) has a history of more than (   ) years.

A. 6000   B. 5000   C. 4000

3. According to TCM theory, the occurrence of diseases is the (   ) between Yin and Yang.

A. correlation   B. incoordination   C. balance

4. In TCM theory, (   ) are the principles of diagnosing and treating diseases.

A. Yin and Yang   B. Wu Xing（五行）   C. Zang-fu viscera （脏腑）

5. (   ) therapy is specially good for pains.

A. moxibustion   B. massage   C. cupping

Vocabulary

acupuncture［ˈækjupʌŋktʃər］*n.* 针灸

pleurapophysis［ˌpluərəˈpɔfisis］*n.*［解剖学］肋突；椎骨侧突

incoordination［ˌɪnkoˌɔrdnˈeʃən］*n.* 不协调

contradictory［ˌkɑ:ntrəˈdɪktəri］*adj.* 相互矛盾的，对立的；*n.* 矛盾命题

moxibustion［ˌmɑ:ksɪˈbʌstʃn］*n.* 艾灸

cupping [ˈkʌpɪŋ] n. 拔火罐

vacuum [ˈvækjuːm] n. 真空；adj. 真空的

Section Ⅱ Speaking

Task 2

You are required to talk about the illustration below in 3 minutes, giving your understanding of methods of processing Chinese Medicinals.

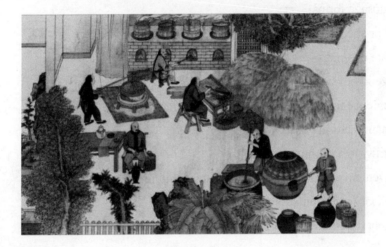

- purifying;
- grinding;
- cutting;
- processing with water;
- processing with fire;
- stir-frying;
- calcining;
- roasting;
- processing with both water and fire;
- other processing methods.

Task 3

Suppose you are working at a pharmaceutical factory, and you are introducing tablets to some visitors. You will answer the questions from them.

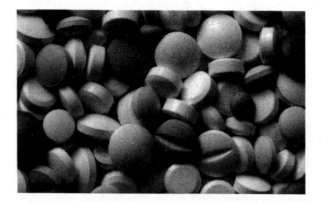

- solid dosage forms;
- round or special-shaped;
- accurate dosing;
- very good physicochemical properties;
- convenience in transportation and administration;
- low manufacturing cost;
- versatility to accommodate;
- inconvenience for swallowing by infants, children and the elderly;
- complexity in formulation and production;
- stringent requirements for quality control.

Section Ⅲ Reading

Medicine

A medicine should make patients better, alleviate symptoms and heal disease—or a combination of all of these—in order to make us healthy. Conventional modern medicine usually involves the use of drug treatment, surgery, counselling or psychological treatment, and lifestyle measure to improve and maintain wellbeing.

Alternative and complementary types of medicine include acupuncture, homeopathy, herbal medicine and traditional Chinese medicines. Not all of these have been proven to be effective, however. Homeopathy, for instance, has been ruled ineffective by the National Health Service in the UK, and British parliamentary committee concluded that homeopathic remedies are not better than placebos.

There is evidence of medical practices, including herbalism—the use of plants for medicinal practices—before the invention of writing and any formally documented history of medicine. Early written records of medicine have been found in ancient Egypt, India and China, as well as the Roman and Greek empires.

The Greek physician Hippocrates is widely credited as the father of modern medicine, and laying the foundation for the conventional approach to medicine. Between the fifth and third centuries BC, Hippocrates introduced the Hippocratic Oath, an ethical vow to do no harm to a patient, which is still invoked by doctors today.

There are concerns that doctors are over-treating people, giving too much medicine and medicalising treatments to people that don't necessarily require medical interventions. Some doctors warn the overzealous use of diagnostic tests and screening programmes can label people with diseases—such as cancer and high blood pressure. Not all of these will be life-threatening or cause health problems, but a diagnosis and medical treatment can cause side effects as well as significant psychological distress.

Task 4

Read the passage and complete the sentences with proper words.

1. A medicine should make patients _____ and heal disease.

2. Alternative and complementary types of medicine include _____ and traditional Chinese medicines.

3. Early written records of medicine have been found in ancient _____.

4. The Greek physician _____ is widely credited as being the father of modern medicine.

5. Hippocrates introduced the _____, an ethical vow to do no harm to a patient, which is still invoked by doctors today.

Task 5

Read the passage and choose the best answer to fill in the blanks.

1. National Health Service in the UK has ruled _____ ineffective.

A. acupuncture

B. psychological treatment

C. homeopathy

D. herbalism

2. Between the_____centuries BC, Hippocrates introduced the Hippocratic Oath.

A. 5&3   B. 4&2   C. 8&4   D. 7&5

3. There are concerns that doctors are over-treating people, giving_____and medicalising treatments to people that don't necessarily require medical interventions.

A. too much health products   B. surgery

C. counselling   D. medicine

Section Ⅳ Writing

Task 6

Suppose you are working at a pharmaceutical company, and you will write an instruction about the preparation of granules. Here are some pictures about granule's production. Discuss with your classmates and write them down.

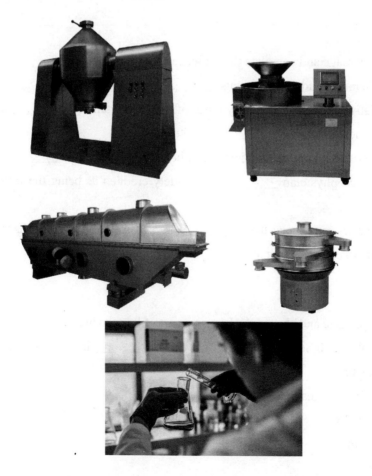

Model 3

Medicine Sale and Management

Unit 8　Insert

Lead-in

The outer label of a drug shall indicate such information as the adopted name in China, ingredients, description, indications or functions, strength, dose and usage, adverse reactions, contraindications, precautions, storage, production date, batch number, expiry date, approval number and manufacturer. Where indications or functions, dose and usage, adverse reactions, contraindications and precautions cannot be fully noted, main information plus a "See drug insert sheet for details" notice shall be indicated.

In-depth Reading

Preview question

What diseases can acetaminophen be used for?

Text

Drug Facts		
Active ingredient (in each tablet)		Purpose
Acetaminophen 325 mg		Pain reliever/fever reducer
Uses		
For the temporary relief of minor aches and pains associated with		
☐ headache　☐ muscular aches　☐ minor arthritis pain　☐ common cold　☐ toothache　☐ dysmenorrhea		
Temporarily reduces fever.		

Warnings

Liver warning: This product contains acetaminophen. Severe liver damage may occur if you take:

☐ more than 4,000 mg in 24 hours, which is the maximum daily amount

☐ with other drugs containing acetaminophen

☐ 3 or more alcoholic drinks every day while using this product

Allergy alert: Acetaminophen may cause severe skin reactions. Symptoms may include:

☐ skin reddening   ☐ blisters   ☐ rash

If a skin reaction occurs, stop use and seek medical help right away.

Do not use

☐ with any other drug containing acetaminophen (prescription or nonprescription). If you are not sure whether a drug contains acetaminophen, ask a doctor or pharmacist.

☐ for more than 10 days for pain unless directed by a doctor

☐ for more than 3 days for fever unless directed by a doctor

Ask a doctor before use if you have

☐ liver disease

Ask a doctor or pharmacist before use if

☐ you are taking the blood thinning drug warfarin

Stop using and ask a doctor if

☐ symptoms do not improve ☐ new symptoms occur

☐ pain or fever persists or gets worse ☐ redness or swelling is present

---

If pregnant or breast-feeding, ask a health professional before use.

Keep out of reach of children. In case of accidental overdose, get medical help or contact a Poison Control Center right away. Prompt medical attention is critical for adults as well as for children even if you do not notice any signs or symptoms.

Directions

☐ do not use more than directed

Adults and children (12 years and older):	Take 2 tablets every 4 to 6 hours as needed. Do not take more than 10 tablets in 24 hours.
Children under 12 years:	Do not give to children under 12 years of age.

Other information

☐ store at room temperature 59-86 ℉ (15-30℃)

☐ tamper-evident sealed packets

☐ do not use any opened or torn packets

Inactive ingredients

corn starch, hypromellose, maltodextrin*, microcrystalline cellulose*, polyethylene glycol, povidone*, pregelatinized starch*, sodium starch glycolate*, stearic acid, titanium dioxide*

* may contain

Questions or comments? Call 1-8xx.234.1464

Vocabulary

acetaminophen [əˌsiːtəˈmɪnəfen] *n.* 对乙酰氨基酚

arthritis [ɑːrˈθraɪtɪs] *n.* 关节炎

allergy [ˈælərdʒi] *n.* 过敏反应，过敏症；厌恶，反感

blister [ˈblɪstər] *n.* [医] 水疱；*v.* 使起水疱

rash [ræʃ] *n.* 皮疹，疹子；一连串（不愉快的事）；*adj.* 轻率的，鲁莽的

pregnant [ˈpregnənt] *adj.* 怀孕的，妊娠的

overdose [ˈoʊvərdoʊs] *n.* 药量过多；（有害物）过量；*v.* 服药过量

prompt [prɑːmpt] *adj.* 迅速的，立刻的；及时的，准时的；*v.* 提示

direction [dəˈrekʃn; daɪˈrekʃn] *n.* 指示，说明；方位；管理，指导

tamper-evident [ˈtæmpə,evidənt] *adj.* （包装）防拆封的；拆封易于被识别的

torn [tɔːrn] *v.* 撕碎，撕裂；撕破，划破；*adj.* 犹豫的

maltodextrin [ˌmæltoʊˈdekstrən] *n.* 麦芽糖糊精

sodium [ˈsoʊdiəm] *n.* 钠（一种化学元素，符号为 Na）；*adj.* 钠光的

Notes

dysmenorrhea 痛经

warfarin 华法林　是一种可以预防中风的血液稀释剂

breast-feeding 母乳喂养

fahrenheit temperature 华氏温度（℉）

celsius temperature 摄氏温度（℃）

hypromellose 羟丙甲纤维素

microcrystalline cellulose 微晶纤维素

polyethylene glycol 聚乙二醇

povidone 聚维酮；聚乙烯吡咯酮

pregelatinized starch 预胶化淀粉

sodium starch glycolate 羟基乙酸淀粉钠；羧甲淀粉钠

stearic acid 硬脂酸

titanium dioxide 二氧化钛

Translation

药品说明	
有效成分（每片）对乙酰氨基酚 325mg	作用类别 镇痛药 / 退烧药

适应证

用于暂时缓解轻至中度疼痛，如

□ 头痛　　□ 肌肉酸痛　　□ 关节疼痛　　□ 感冒　　□ 牙痛　　□ 痛经

暂时减少发热。

警告

肝损伤警告：本品含有对乙酰氨基酚。如果在以下情况时服用，可能会造成严重的肝脏损伤：

□ 24 小时内超过 4000mg，这是一天的最大摄入量

□ 和其他含有对乙酰氨基酚的药物一起服用

□ 使用本产品时，每天饮用 3 杯或 3 杯以上的酒精饮料

过敏警示：对乙酰氨基酚可能引起严重的皮肤反应。症状可能包括：

□ 皮肤变红　　□ 水疱　　□ 皮疹

如果出现皮肤反应，立即停止使用并寻求医疗帮助。

请勿使用

□ 正在服用任何其他含有对乙酰氨基酚的药物（处方或非处方）。如果你不确定药物中是否含有对乙酰氨基酚，请咨询医生或药剂师。

□ 疼痛超过 10 天，除非是在医生指导之下

□ 发烧超过 3 天，除非是在医生指导之下

如果有以下情况，请在使用前咨询医生

□ 肝病

如果有以下情况，请在使用前咨询医生或药剂师

□ 正在服用血液稀释药华法林

如果有以下情况，停止使用并咨询医生

□ 症状没有改善　　□ 出现新的症状　　□ 持续疼痛或发烧，或恶化　　□ 出现红肿

妊娠期或哺乳期，请在使用前咨询健康专家。

放置在儿童接触不到的地方。如果意外服用过量，即使你没有观察到任何迹象或症状，也应立即寻求医疗帮助或联系毒物控制中心。及时就医对成人和儿童都至关重要。

用法用量

□ 不要超过指导用量

成人和儿童：（12 岁及以上）	根据需要，每 4 ～ 6 小时服用 2 片。24 小时内服用的药片不要超过 10 片。
12 岁以下儿童：	不要给 12 岁以下的儿童服用。

其他信息

□ 在室温 59 ～ 86°F（15 ～ 30℃）下储存

□ 防拆封的密封包装

□ 包装损坏，不要使用

非活性成分

玉米淀粉、羟丙甲纤维素、麦芽糊精 *、微晶纤维素 *、聚乙二醇、聚维酮 *、预胶化淀粉 *、羟基乙酸淀粉钠 *、硬脂酸、二氧化钛 *

"*" 表示可能含有

如有什么问题或意见？请拨打 1-8xx.234.1464

Quiz

I. Answer the questions according to the text.

1. What diseases can acetaminophen be used for?

_____

2. If blisters appear, can the patient continue to take acetaminophen?

_____

3. Is hypromellose an active ingredient?

_____

4. Can anyone over the age of 12 take this medicine ?

_____

II. Complete the sentences with the words given. Change the form if necessary.

liver	torn	prompt	rash
sodium	reach	breast-feeding	allergy

1. In theory, any food can cause an _____.
2. There are many emergencies which need _____ first aid treatment.
3. He suffered _____ ligaments in his knee.
4. Some women find _____ logistically difficult because of work.
5. Common salt is a compound of _____ and chlorine.
6. The heat brought him out in a _____ .
7. The largest organ in the body is the _____ .
8. Victory is now out of her _____ .

III. Translation between English and Chinese.

muscular ache	活性成分
menstrual cramp	关节疼痛
inactive ingredient	室温
breast-feeding	密封包装

Extended Reading

Text

Provisions for Drug Insert Sheets and Labels

Chapter II Drug Insert Sheet

Article 9　A drug insert sheet shall include the significant scientific data, conclusions and information concerning drug safety and efficacy in order to direct the safe and rational use of drugs. The specific format, content and writing requirements of drug insert sheet shall be prescribed and issued by the State Food and Drug Administration.

Article 10　Disease names, pharmaceutical terms, drug names, the names and results of clinical testing in drug insert sheets shall be expressed in professional terms published or standardized by the State. The units of measurement shall conform to the national standards.

Article 11　All the active ingredients or medicinal ingredients of traditional Chinese medicines in a prescription shall be listed in the insert sheet. For injections and non-prescription drugs, all excipients shall be listed as well.

The ingredients or excipients included in a prescription, which may cause severe adverse reaction, shall be specified.

Article 12　A drug manufacturer shall trace the safety and efficacy of its marketed drugs. For any modification to the insert sheet, an application shall be submitted timely.

The State Food and Drug Administration may also require a drug manufacturer to make modification to the insert sheet on the basis of the results of adverse drug reaction monitoring and drug re-evaluation.

Article 13　After the modification to the insert sheet is approved, the drug manufacturer shall inform relevant drug distributors, drug users and other departments of the modified content immediately, and use the modified insert sheet and label timely as required.

Article 14　The insert sheet shall provide full information on adverse drug reaction and indicate the adverse reactions in detail. A drug manufacturer, who fails to timely modify the insert sheet on the basis of the safety and efficacy data of the marketed drug or to fully explain the adverse reaction in the insert sheet, shall be liable for all the consequences arising therefrom.

Article 15　The approval date and the modification date shall be distinctively shown in the insert sheet.

Vocabulary

insert [ɪnˈsɜːrt] n. 插入物；插页，附加页；v. 插入，嵌入
sheet [ʃiːt] n. 纸片，纸张；工作表；床单，被单；纪要
rational [ˈræʃnəl] adj. 合理的；理性的，理智的；（数）有理数的；n. 有理数
excipient [ɪkˈsɪpɪənt] n. ［药］辅料

trace [treɪs] *v.* 查出，发现，追踪；追溯，追究；*n.* 痕迹，遗迹，踪迹

efficacy [ˈefɪkəsi] *n.* 功效，效力

modification [ˌmɑːdɪfɪˈkeɪʃn] *n.* 修改的行为（过程）；修改，更改；修饰

consequence [ˈkɑːnsɪkwens] *n.* 结果，后果；重要性，价值

distinctively [dɪˈstɪŋktɪvli] *adv.* 特殊地；区别地

Translation

药品说明书和标签管理规定

第二章　药品说明书

第九条　药品说明书应当包含药品安全性、有效性的重要科学数据、结论和信息，用以指导安全、合理使用药品。药品说明书的具体格式、内容和书写要求由国家食品药品监督管理局制定并发布。

第十条　药品说明书对疾病名称、药学专业名词、药品名称、临床检验名称和结果的表述，应当采用国家统一颁布或规范的专用词汇，度量衡单位应当符合国家标准的规定。

第十一条　药品说明书应当列出全部活性成分或者组方中的全部中药药味。注射剂和非处方药还应当列出所用的全部辅料名称。

药品处方中含有可能引起严重不良反应的成分或者辅料的，应当予以说明。

第十二条　药品生产企业应当主动跟踪药品上市后的安全性、有效性情况，需要对药品说明书进行修改的，应当及时提出申请。

根据药品不良反应监测、药品再评价结果等信息，国家食品药品监督管理局也可以要求药品生产企业修改药品说明书。

第十三条　药品说明书获准修改后，药品生产企业应当将修改的内容立即通知相关药品经营企业、使用单位及其他部门，并按要求及时使用修改后的说明书和标签。

第十四条　药品说明书应当充分包含药品不良反应信息，详细注明药品不良反应。药品生产企业未根据药品上市后的安全性、有效性情况及时修改说明书或者未将药品不良反应在说明书中充分说明的，由此引起的不良后果由该生产企业承担。

第十五条　药品说明书核准日期和修改日期应当在说明书中醒目标示。

......

Unit 9　Medicine Sale

Lead-in

When a salesperson understands the buyer, he can provide the buyer with what they want & when they want. For example, your buyer needs a trial to evaluate your product but can't allocate more than 30 minutes to it, give them a free trial that is easy to set up, easy to use and demonstrates the value of your product in five minutes or less.

In-depth Reading

Preview questions

    1. Under what conditions, must the patient stop taking the drug immediately? (Dialogue 1)

    2. Can this medicine lower blood pressure? (Dialogue 2)

Text

Dialogue 1

（Pharmacist:P; Customer:C）

P:Good morning sir, what can I do for you?

C:Here is the prescription the doctor gave me, could you please fetch these medicines for me?

P:Oh,let me have a look, this may take a few minutes.

(A moment later)

P:OK sir, your prescription is all set, what the doctor wrote is a medication to help you sleep, and you may take them one time a day, 1 pill a time, about 2 or 3 hours before going to sleep. Please remember that do not take them together with alcohol. Just be careful, sometimes when you wake up in the morning you may feel a little bit hangover or drowsy.

C:Oh, really, you mean hangover like after getting drunk the night before?

P:Yes, but don't worry about it, this is the normal side effect of the medicine. You'd better not drive if you feel quite drowsy which can be quite dangerous. But if this feeling gets especially strong, you should stop using this medicine and go to see the doctor.

C:Oh, I see, thanks a lot. Is there any other thing that I need to pay attention to?

P:Some people might be allergic to this medicine. So if you have rash on your skin or your eye white become yellow, you should also stop using it immediately and consult the doctor as soon as you can.

C:Hopefully that terrible stuff won't happen on me, thank you very much.

P:You are welcome, have a nice day.

Dialogue 2

(Medical Representative:MR; Doctor:D)

MR:This drug has been clinically observed by the first hospital, the second hospital of Medical University, the X Province Institute of Traditional Chinese drug, and other institutions. The total clinical effective rate is 94% after taking 30 days.Routine laboratory tests of blood, urine, and stool, and liver and kidney function tests showed no adverse reactions.

D:Every sales representative said this to me, so let's be practical!

MR:This medicine can significantly reduce hyperglycemia, and has no effect on normal blood sugar, so there will be no hypoglycemia reaction. It can significantly reduce blood lipids, especially lower the triglycerides.

D:Sounds great. Are there any other features?

MR:It can significantly reduce serum lipid peroxides, and it has the effects of anti-oxidation and protection of the body. In addition it is of great benefit to the prevention and treatment of diabetes complications.

D:Diabetes patients often have complications. If this medicine is really like what you said, it would be fine!

MR:Do you want to try?

D:What is the dose? What should patients pay attention to when taking it?

MR:They need to control their diet during the medication. No smoking, no alcohol, and no spicy. 30 days is a course of treatment, and it is recommended to take no less than 3 to 6 courses of treatment continuously.

Vocabulary

dialogue ['daɪəlɔːg] *n.* 对白；对话，交换意见；*v.* 参加对话，进行讨论

hangover ['hæŋouvər] *n.* 宿醉；残留物；遗物

drowsy ['drauzi] *adj.* 昏昏欲睡的，困倦的；令人松弛的，令人困倦欲睡的；（尤指地方）静谧的，平静的，安静的

stuff [stʌf] *n.* 活动，事情；东西，物品；基本特征，特质，根本

representative [ˌreprɪ'zentətɪv] *n.* 代表

institute ['ɪnstɪtuːt] *n.* 研究所，学院，协会

urine ['jʊrɪn] *n.* 尿液，小便

stool [stuːl] *n.* 大便，粪便；凳子；（生长新芽的）根株，母株；厕所

practical ['præktɪkl] *adj.* 真实的，实际的；切实有效的，切实可行的

hyperglycemia [ˌhaɪpərglaɪ'siːmɪə] *n.* 高血糖症

lipid ['lɪpɪd] *n.* 脂质；油脂

triglyceride [traɪ'glɪsəraɪd] *n.* 三酰甘油；甘油三酯

serum ['sɪrəm] *n.* 血清；免疫血清；（植物的）浆液，树液

peroxide [pə'rɑːksaɪd] *n.* 过氧化氢；过氧化物

Notes

hypnotic　催眠药

fill in　填写；填充；临时代替；填满

anti-oxidation　抗氧化

Translation

对话 1

（药剂师：P；客户：C）

P：早上好，先生，有什么可以帮助您的吗？

C：这是医生给我开的处方，能帮我拿一下药吗？

P：让我看看，请稍等。

（片刻之后）

P：好的，先生，您的药已经准备好了，医生开的是一种帮助您睡眠的药物，您可以每天服用一次，每次一片，在睡觉前 2～3 小时服用。请记住，不要与酒精一起

服用，还有就是，当您早上醒来时，您可能会有宿醉或者昏昏欲睡的感觉。

C：真的？是像前一天晚上喝醉后的宿醉？

P：是的，但是别担心，这是药物的正常副作用。如果您感到昏昏欲睡，最好不要开车，这很危险。但是如果这种感觉特别强烈的话，建议您停止使用这种药，去看医生。

C：我明白了，非常感谢，还有什么需要我注意的吗？

P：有些人可能对这种药过敏，所以如果您的皮肤出现皮疹或眼白变黄，您也应该立即停止使用，并尽快咨询医生。

C：非常感谢，希望这些糟糕的事情不会发生在我身上。

P：不客气，祝您有个美好的一天。

对话 2

（医药代表：MR；医生：D）

MR：该药已在医科大学第一医院、第二医院、X 省中药研究所等机构进行临床观察。服用 30 天后，临床有效率为 94%。血液、尿液、粪便和肝肾功能的常规实验室检查均未发现不良反应。

D：每个医药代表都这么对我说，请实际客观一点！

MR：该药能显著降低高血糖，对正常血糖无影响，不会出现低血糖反应。它能显著降血脂，尤其是甘油三酯。

D：听起来不错，还有其他优点吗？

MR：它能显著降低血清脂质过氧化物，具有抗氧化作用，对糖尿病并发症的预防和治疗有很大益处。

D：糖尿病患者经常有并发症。这种药如果真的像您说的那样，那就好了！

MR：您要考虑一下吗？

D：剂量是多少？患者服用时应注意什么？

MR：30 天为一个疗程，建议连续服用不少于 3 ～ 6 个疗程。服药期间控制饮食、不吸烟、不喝酒、忌辛辣。

Quiz

Ⅰ. Answer the questions according to the text.

1. Under what conditions, must the patient stop taking the drug immediately? （Dialogue 1）

_____

2. What medicine did the customer buy ？ （Dialogue 1）

_____

3. Can this medicine lower blood pressure?（Dialogue 2）

_____

4. Why did doctor let medical representative be practical?（Dialogue 2）

_____

Ⅱ. Complete the sentences with the words given. Change the form if necessary.

drowsy	hypnotics	stuff	representative
peroxide	hangover	urine	lipid

1. Certain drugs such as benzodiazepines, which are tranquillisers and _____.

2. I felt dopey and _____ after the operation.

3. Soybean is the main source of plant protein and _____ for mankind.

4. The doctor took a _____ sample and a blood sample.

5. The painting is not _____ of his work of the period.

6. He woke up with a terrible _____ .

7. If we take hydrogen _____ in the liquid state, it can break down to form water and oxygen.

8. I called Andie to tell her how spectacular the _____ looked.

Ⅲ. Translation between English and Chinese.

Medical Representative	糖尿病
blood sugar	催眠药
kidney function	困倦的
hypoglycemia reaction	

Extended Reading

Text

7 Skills Every Salesperson Should Master

No. 1: Understand what the buyer wants

Understanding the buyer is the foundation of effective selling, but it involves more than just knowing who the buyer is. Instead, it's about identifying the experience the buyer wants to have as they consider making a purchase in your market.

Your buyer has a set of expectations about that experience and your job as a salesperson is to exceed those expectations. You can't exceed them if you don't understand the experience that the buyer wants to have.

No. 2: Use psychology to engage the buyer

There are a variety of psychological techniques you can use to create deeper engagement with your target buyers. One effective tip is to make sure that the customer knows you won't take too much of their time.

No. 3: Establish trust with the buyer

Buyers like to do business with people they trust. Good salespeople view their ability to establish trust with the buyer as a core sales skill.

No. 4: Communicate succinctly

Buyers often value how information is presented more than the information itself. A good rule is to never try to communicate more than three important points in a single conversation with a buyer.

No. 5: Act on what the customer is saying

The best salespeople take action based on what they hear from their customer. It's not good enough to just listen—you need to internalize what the buyer has said and then do something about it.

No. 6: Demonstrate subject matter expertise

Salespeople need to understand the buyer, the pressing issues the buyer is facing and what they want as they work their way to a purchase. They also need to have expertise about their own product or service and the industry.

No. 7: Tell compelling stories

Buyers don't really want to hear about your product or service. Good salespeople know this and weave the product or service they're selling into a larger story that has an arc and ends with the customer receiving what they want, which is usually not your product.

Vocabulary

master ['mæstər] v. 精通；控制；征服；n. 硕士；主人；大师

foundation [faʊn'deɪʃn] n. 基础；基本原理；基金会；建立，创办；粉底霜

involve [ɪn'vɑːlv] v. 涉及，牵涉；包含，需要

purchase ['pɜːrtʃəs] n. 购买，采购

engage [ɪn'geɪdʒ] v. 吸引，引起；雇用，聘请；参加，从事

demonstrate ['demənstreɪt] v. 证明；示范，演示；表露；游行，示威

expertise [ˌekspɜːrˈtiːz] *n.* 专长，专门技能（知识）；专家的意见

industry [ˈɪndəstri] *n.* 行业，产业；勤奋，勤劳；范围，领域

compelling [kəmˈpelɪŋ] *adj.* 令人信服的，有说服力的；引人入胜的，扣人心弦的

Translation

每个销售人员都应该掌握的 7 项技能

No.1：了解买家想要什么

了解买方是有效销售的基础，不仅需要知道买方是谁，还要了解他们购买你的产品时想要拥有的体验。

买家对这种体验有一系列期望，而作为销售人员，你的工作就是尽可能满足这些期望。如果你不了解买家想要的体验，你就无法满足他们。

No.2：利用心理学吸引买家

您可以使用各种心理技巧与目标买家建立更深入的互动。友情提示：需要让客户知道您不会花费他们太多的时间。

No.3：与买方建立信任

买家喜欢与他们信任的人做生意。优秀的销售人员需要把与买家建立信任的能力视为核心销售技能。

No.4：简明扼要地沟通

购买者通常更看重信息的呈现方式，而不是信息本身。有效方法是：在与买家的一次对话中，传递的信息要点尽量不超过三个。

No.5：根据客户的意愿采取行动

优秀的销售人员可以根据他们从客户那里听到的信息采取行动。仅仅倾听是不够的，您需要内化买家所说的话，然后对此做出反应。

No.6：展示专业知识与技能

销售人员需要了解买家，包括买家面临的紧迫问题以及他们在购买过程中想要什么。除此外，他们还需要具备自己的产品或服务以及行业相关的专业知识。

No.7：讲述引人入胜的故事

有时买家对您的产品或服务并不感兴趣。优秀的销售人员知道这一点后，将他们销售的产品或服务隐含在一个故事中，这个故事应该是围绕购买者的需求展开，而不是您的产品。

Unit 10　Drug Administration

Lead-in

Storing your medicine：

① Keep medicines in their original containers and in a cool, dry place. Although people may think the bathroom cabinet is a good storage place, it is usually too hot and humid;

② Follow any special storage instructions: Some medicines should be refrigerated;

③ Store medicines out of the reach and sight of children. If there are children in the home, use the child-resistant caps.

In-depth Reading

Preview question

Why patients should know Pradaxa storage precautions ?

Text

Special Storage and Handling Requirements Must Be Followed

for Pradaxa Capsules

Pradaxa is an anticoagulant (or blood thinner) medication known as a direct thrombin inhibitor. It works by preventing the formation of blood clots，and is used to prevent strokes or serious blood clots in people who have non-valvular atrial fibrillation (irregular heart beat).

Many consumers use pill boxes or pill organizers to aid them in remembering to take their medications. However, because of the potential for product breakdown and loss of potency, consumers should not store Pradaxa in any container other than the original manufacturer packaging. Additionally, pharmacists should only dispense Pradaxa capsules in the original manufacturer packaging. Using the manufacturer packaging will minimize product breakdown from moisture. Pradaxa is packaged in a bottle containing a 30-day supply with a desiccant (drying agent) in the cap to keep moisture away from the capsules. Pradaxa capsules are also available in a blister package which protects from moisture.

1. Additional information for patients

(1) Store Pradaxa in the original bottle or blister package to protect from moisture.

(2) Do not store or place Pradaxa capsules in any other container, such as pill boxes or pill organizers.

(3) For Pradaxa bottles:

① Open only one bottle of Pradaxa at a time. Once the bottle is opened, the product must be used within 60 days.

② Remove only one capsule from the bottle at the time of use. The bottle should be immediately closed tightly.

③ Date the bottle to expire 60 days after opening.

(4) For Pradaxa blister packages:Open the blister package at time of use. Do not open or puncture the blister earlier than the time of use.

(5) Discuss any questions or concerns about Pradaxa with your healthcare professional.

(6) Read the Medication Guide for Pradaxa each time you get your prescription refilled.

(7) Report any side effects you experience to the FDA MedWatch program using the information in the "Contact Us" box at the bottom of the page.

2. Additional information for healthcare professionals

(1) Tell patients it is important to follow the special storage and handling requirements for Pradaxa.

(2) Tell patients that Pradaxa must be kept in the original bottle or blister package to protect from moisture. The bottle contains a dessicant in the cap and the blister package protects unopened pills from moisture.

(3) Tell patients that Pradaxa capsules could not be stored in pill boxes or pill organizers.

(4) Pharmacists should only dispense Pradaxa in the original manufacturer bottle with the original dessicant cap. Do not repackage Pradaxa capsules in standard amber pharmacy vials.

(5) Pharmacists should not open the Pradaxa bottle when dispensing. When more than one bottle is dispensed, tell the patient to only open one bottle at a time.

(6) Pharmacists should place an auxiliary expiration label on the bottle and instruct the patients to date the bottle to expire 60 days after opening.

(7) Pharmacists can also number the bottles (e.g., bottle 1$^{#}$ and bottle 2$^{#}$) when dispensing multiple bottles so the patient can keep track of which bottle they opened.

(8) Report adverse events involving Pradaxa to the FDA MedWatch program, using the information in the "Contact Us" box at the bottom of the page.

FDA is concerned that these special storage and handling requirements are not commonly known and are not being followed by Pradaxa users and pharmacies. Boehringer Ingelheim Pharmaceuticals, Inc., the manufacturer of Pradaxa, has started a campaign to educate healthcare professionals (prescribers and pharmacists) about these requirements. FDA is emphasizing that healthcare professionals must also reinforce the importance of these special storage and handling requirements to their patients.

Vocabulary

anticoagulant [ˌæntikoʊˈægjələnt] *n.* 抗凝血剂；*adj.* 抗凝血的

thrombin [ˈθrɑːmbɪn] *n.* 凝血酶

inhibitor [ɪnˈhɪbɪtər] *n.* 抑制剂，抑制因素；抑制者

clot [klɑːt] *n.* 凝块（尤指血块）；*v.* （使）凝结成块

stroke [stroʊk] *n.* 中风

potency [ˈpoʊtnsi] *n.* （药物等的）效力；影响力，支配力

dispense [dɪˈspens] *v.* 配发（药）；发放，分配；提供，施予

minimize [ˈmɪnɪmaɪz] *v.* 使减少到最低限度；（在计算机屏幕上）使最小化

moisture [ˈmɔɪstʃər] *n.* 潮气，水分

desiccant [ˈdesɪkənt] *n.* 干燥剂；*adj.* 去湿的，使干燥的

puncture [ˈpʌŋktʃər] *v.* 刺破，戳破；*n.* （被尖物刺穿的）小洞

auxiliary [ɔːgˈzɪliəri] *adj.* 辅助的；备用的；*n.* 助手，辅助人员

emphasize [ˈemfəsaɪz] *v.* 强调，着重；重读；使突出

reinforce [ˌriːɪnˈfɔːrs] *v.* 加强，强化；加固；寻求增援；*n.* 加固物

Notes

Pradaxa 泰毕全　前沿的新一代口服抗凝血药、直接凝血酶抑制剂，用于预防非瓣膜性房颤患者的脑卒中和全身性血液凝固。

blood clot 血凝块，血栓

non-valvular atrial fibrillation (NVAF) 非瓣膜性房颤

Translation

泰毕全胶囊特殊的储存和处理要求

泰毕全是一种抗凝血剂（或血液稀释剂），被称为直接凝血酶抑制剂。它的药理作用是防止血栓形成，用于预防患有非瓣膜性房颤（不规则心跳）患者的中风或严重血栓。

许多患者使用分药盒来帮助他们服药。然而，分药盒可能会导致药物分解和失去药效，患者不应将泰毕全储存在除原包装外的其他任何容器中。此外，药剂师应仅以生产厂家的原始包装分发泰毕全胶囊。使用原包装将最大限度地避免药物因受潮而分解。将 30 天药量的泰毕全封装在一个瓶中，瓶盖中含有干燥剂，以保持药品干燥。泰毕全胶囊的泡罩包装也可以起到防潮作用。

1. 为患者提供的信息

（1）将泰毕全储存在原装瓶或泡罩包装中，以防受潮。

（2）不要将泰毕全胶囊储存或放置在其他任何容器中，如药箱或分药盒。

（3）关于泰毕全的药瓶：

① 一次只打开一瓶。一旦开封，必须在 60 天内使用。

② 使用时只从药瓶中取出一粒胶囊，并立即盖紧瓶盖。

③ 药瓶在打开 60 天后过期。

（4）关于泰毕全的泡罩包装：仅在使用时打开泡罩包装。不要在使用之前打开或刺穿泡罩。

（5）与医生或健康顾问反馈有关泰毕全的任何问题或担忧。

（6）每次重新用药都要阅读泰毕全的用药指南。

（7）使用页面底部"联系我们"框中的信息，向 FDA MedWatch 计划报告遇到的任何副作用。

2. 为医疗专业人员提供的信息

（1）告诉患者遵守泰毕全的特殊储存和处理要求很重要。

（2）告诉患者，泰毕全必须保存在原装瓶或泡罩包装中，以防受潮。瓶中装有干燥剂，泡罩包装可防止未打开的药丸受潮。

（3）告诉患者，泰毕全胶囊不得存放在药箱或分药盒中。

（4）药剂师应只配发装在原装瓶中的泰毕全胶囊，因为原装瓶带有原装干燥剂瓶盖。不要将泰毕全胶囊重新分装在棕色药瓶中。

（5）发药时，药剂师不要打开泰毕全原装瓶。当配药超过一瓶时，告诉患者一次只打开一瓶。

（6）药剂师应在瓶身贴上一个日期标签，提示患者药瓶在打开后 60 天过期。

（7）药剂师还可以在分发多瓶泰毕全时对药瓶（例如，瓶 1 和瓶 2）进行编号，以便患者清楚区分出他们打开的药瓶。

（8）使用页面底部"联系我们"框中的信息，向 FDA MedWatch 计划报告涉及泰毕全的不良事件。

FDA 担心这些特殊的储存和处理要求并没有广为人知，泰毕全使用者和药房无法遵守这些要求。泰毕全的制造商勃林格·殷格翰制药有限公司发起了一场运动，就这些特殊要求对医疗专业人员（处方师和药剂师）进行培训。FDA 建议，医疗专业人员必须向患者强调遵守这些特殊储存和处理要求的重要性。

Quiz

I. Answer the questions according to the text.

1. Why patients should know Pradaxa storage precautions ?

_____

2. How to store Pradaxa ?

_____

3. Does Pradaxa bottle expire after 60 hours after opening?

_____

4. Can Pradaxa help clot formation?

_____

II. Complete the sentences with the words given. Change the form if necessary.

potency	clot	anticoagulant	minimize
moisture	strokes	emphasize	desiccant

1. My skin feels tight and lacking in _____ .

2. I tried to _____ my good points without sounding boastful.

3. If you keep a medicine too long, it may lose its _____ .

4. Good hygiene helps to _____ the risk of infection.

5. His blood was normal. They could find no reason for the _____.

6. Many doctors, including me, would advise you to take an _____ such as warfarin indefinitely.

7. These goods are susceptible to water, remember to add a _____ when you store them.

8. The most common of the serious emergencies include heart trouble, _____, and difficulty breathing.

Ⅲ. Translation between English and Chinese.

blood clot   泡罩包装

healthcare professional   储存要求

irregular heart beat   切勿受潮

Extended Reading

Text

How to Store Household Medicines

(1) Store in refrigeration. All medicines that will deteriorate or deform due to high temperature should be stored in a low temperature environment. Generally, the room temperature cannot meet this requirement, so they should be kept in the refrigerator. The storage temperature of medicines is generally indicated on the packaging. Commonly used are insulin, gamma globulin and various biological preparations, and medicines that are easily deformed after heating include various anal suppositories and vaginal suppositories.

(2) Keep tightly closed. Some medicines are prone to weathering when left in the air for a long time and should be kept tightly closed, such as borax, magnesium sulfate, citric acid, etc. ; some medicines will be oxidized when exposed to air for a long time, such as vitamin C, cod liver oil drops, etc. Some volatile drugs, such as safflower oil, iodine and other alcohol-containing preparations, should also be kept tightly closed. The medicines to be kept tightly closed should be placed in glass bottles with the mouth of the bottle tightly sealed and cannot be stored in a paper box, otherwise they will deteriorate.

(3) Store in moisture-proof. Many medicines will absorb moisture in the air and be deliquescent in humid air. The medicines may be deliquescence, such as melting, moldy, fermentation, adhesion, etc., so these medicines cannot be used. Therefore, you should try to put them in airtight vials and store them in a dry place. Drugs that are particularly prone to deliquesce include: aspirin, dry yeast, vitamin B_1, calcium gluconate, and some sugar-coated tablets, and capsules are also very susceptible to moisture.

(4) Store in the dark. Some medicines such as aminophylline, vitamin C, nitroglycerin

and various injections will deteriorate under the action of light. They should be placed in a brown bottle and stored in a dark place. Of course, other drugs should be protected from light as much as possible.

Vocabulary

refrigeration [rɪˌfrɪdʒəˈreɪʃn] *n.* 冷藏，冷冻

deteriorate [dɪˈtɪrɪəreɪt] *v.* 恶化，变坏

deform [dɪˈfɔːrm] *v.* 改变……的外形，损毁……的形状

borax [ˈbɔːræks] *n.* 硼砂

magnesium [mægˈniːziəm] *n.* 镁

sulfate [ˈsʌlfeɪt] *n.* 硫酸盐；*v.* 使成硫酸盐；用硫酸处理

oxidize [ˈɑːksɪdaɪz] *v.* 使氧化；使生锈；氧化

volatile [ˈvɑːlətl] *adj.* 易变的；（液体或固体）易挥发的；*n.* 挥发物

iodine [ˈaɪədaɪn] *n.* 碘；碘酒

deliquesce [ˌdelɪˈkwes] *v.* 潮解，溶解；液化

moldy [ˈmoʊldi] *adj.* 发霉的；乏味的；陈腐的

adhesion [ædˈhiːʒn] *n.* 附着；黏附（力）；支持；固定

aminophylline [əˌmiːnoʊˈfɪlain] *n.* 氨茶碱

nitroglycerin [ˌnaɪtroʊˈɡlɪsərɪn] *n.* 硝酸甘油；三硝酸甘油酯

Notes

gamma globulin   丙种球蛋白；γ 球蛋白
safflower oil   红花油

Translation

如何妥善储存各类家用药品

（1）冷藏保存   凡温度过高会变质或变形的药品应放在低温环境中保存，一般室温达不到这一要求，因此宜放在冰箱中冷藏。受热后易变质的药品一般都会在包装上注明贮藏温度，常用的有胰岛素、丙种球蛋白及各种生物制剂。受热后易变形的药品有各种肛门栓剂、阴道栓剂。

（2）密闭保存   有些药品久置空气中易风化，应密闭保存，如硼砂、硫酸镁、枸橼酸等。有些药品长期接触空气会被氧化，如维生素 C、鱼肝油滴剂等。一些易挥发的药物，如红花油、碘酒及其他含酒精的制剂也要密闭保存。要密闭保存的药物应放

在玻璃瓶内，瓶口要封严，不能用纸盒贮存，否则易变质。

（3）防潮保存　许多药品在潮湿的空气中，会吸收空气中的水分而潮解，药品出现融化、发霉、发酵、粘连等潮解现象后就不能使用。因此，应尽量将这类药品放在密闭的容器内，并置于干燥处保存。特别容易潮解的药品有：阿司匹林、干酵母、维生素 B_1、葡萄糖酸钙及一些含糖多的糖衣片，胶囊剂也极易受潮。

（4）避光保存　有些药品如氨茶碱、维生素 C、硝酸甘油及各种针剂在光线作用下易变质，应放置在棕色瓶中并置于暗处保存。当然，其他药品也要尽量避光。

Mini Project 3

Section Ⅰ Listening

A patient and a chemist are talking about common drugs. Listen carefully, and complete Task 1.

Task 1

1. Which of the following is true? (   )

A. The patient has a toothache.

B. The patient has a headache.

C. The patient has a muscular ache.

2. Is the patient allergic to any type of medication? (   )

A. He is allergic to penicillin.

B. He isn't allergic to any type of medication.

C. He doesn't know exactly.

3. Why can't the patient buy penicillin? (   )

A. He didn't get a doctor's prescription.

B. He is allergic to penicillin.

C. The pharmacist didn't want to sell it.

4. What medicine did the patient buy? (   )

A. boric acid and cough syrup

B. amoxicillin and cough syrup

C. penicillin and cough syrup

5. What's the best drink for this patient? (   )

A. ice water

B. cola

C. hot tea along with some honey

Vocabulary

boric acid　硼酸

syrup ['sɪrəp] *n.* 糖浆

lozenge['lɑːzɪndʒ] *n.* 锭剂

Section Ⅱ Speaking

Task 2

You are required to talk about the illustration in 3 minutes, giving your understanding of the information of the drug in the illustration.

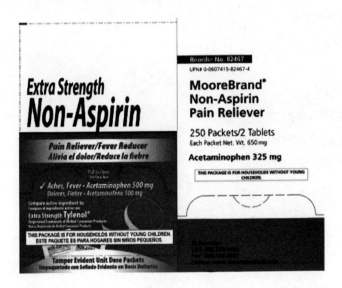

• reliever;

• acetaminophen;

• reorder;

• household;

• package;

• net wt.

Task 3

Suppose you are working at a drugstore, and you are introducing products to some customers. You will answer the questions from them.

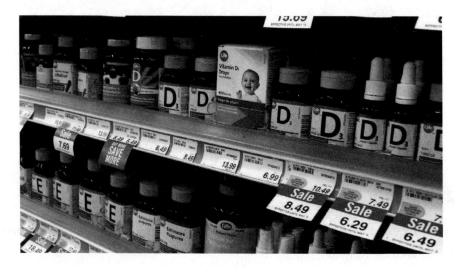

- melatonin tablet;
- soft capsule;
- calcium;
- mineral;
- improving sleeping ;
- improving gastrointestinal functions;
- relaxing bowel.

Section Ⅲ Reading

How to Dispose of Medicines at Home

When a take-back option is not easily available, there are two ways to dispose of medicines at home depending on the drug.

Flushing medicines: Because some medicines could be especially harmful to others, there are specific directions to immediately flush them down the sink or toilet when they are no longer needed, and a take-back option is not readily available.

How will you know? Check the label or the patient information leaflet with your medicine. Or consult the U.S. Food and Drug Administration's list of medicines recommended for disposal by flushing when a take-back option is not readily available. Remember, don't flush your medicine unless it is on the flush list.

Disposing medicines in household trash: If a take-back program is not available, almost all medicines, except those on the FDA flush list, can be thrown into your household trash. These include prescription and over-the-counter (OTC) drugs in pills, liquids, drops, patches, and creams.

Follow these steps:

(1) Remove the drugs from their original containers and mix them with something undesirable, such as used coffee grounds, dirt, or cat litter. This makes the medicine less appealing to children and pets and unrecognizable to someone who might intentionally go through the trash looking for drugs.

(2) Put the mixture in something you can close (a re-sealable zipper storage bag, empty can, or other container) to prevent the drug from leaking or spilling out.

(3) Throw the container in the garbage.

(4) Scratch out all your personal information on the empty medicine packaging to protect your identity and privacy. Throw the packaging away.

If you have a question about your medicine, ask your healthcare provider or pharmacist.

Task 4

Read the passage and complete the sentences with proper words.

1.When a take-back option is not easily available, there are two ways to _____ of medicines at home.

2. Some medicines could be especially _____ to others.

3. Check the _____ or the patient information leaflet with your medicine.

4. Put the mixture in something you can close to _____ the drug from leaking or spilling out.

5. Remove the drugs from their original _____.

Task 5

Read the passage and choose the best answer to fill in the blanks.

1. What is this article talking about? (   )

A. How to dispose of medicines at home.

B. How to store medicines at home.

C. How to dispose of medicines at hospital.

D. How to store medicines at hospital.

2. How many ways to dispose drugs are mentioned in the article? (　　)

A. 3   B. 2   C. 1   D. 5

3. Why do some drugs need to be flushed into the sink or toilet ? (　　)

A. Because they are harmless to others.

B. Because they can't mix with cat litter.

C. Because they can pollute the air.

D. Because they are harmful to others.

Section Ⅳ Writing

Task 6

Suppose you are working at a pharmaceutical company, and you will write an introduction to the product. Here are some pictures about the product. Discuss with your classmates and write them down.

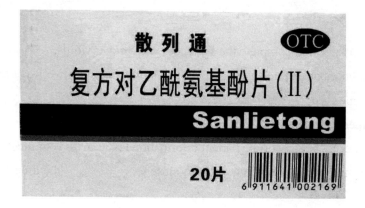

References

［1］　Constitution of the World Health Organization. Basic Documents, Forty-fifth edition, Supplement, ［2006.10］.

［2］　COVID-19: Symptoms, Prevention and Risks. ［2021.11.30］. https://www.drugs.com/article/covid-19-symptoms-prevention.html.

［3］　Wikipedia. Drug. ［2021.10.21］. http://en.volupedia.org/wiki/Drug.

［4］　Managing Common Drug Side Effects. ［2020.11.23］. https://www.drugs.com/article/drug-side-effects.html.

［5］　Wikipedia. Antibiotic. ［2021.12.15］. http://en.volupedia.org/wiki/Antibiotic.

［6］　Nonsteroidal anti-inflammatory drugs. ［2018.3.22］. https://www.drugs.com/drug-class/nonsteroidal-anti-inflammatory-agents.html.

［7］　滕佳林. 中药学. 2 版. 北京：人民卫生出版社，2019.

［8］　Good manufacturing practice for drugs(2010 version). National medical products administration. 2010.

［9］　卫生部. 药品生产质量管理规范. 北京：2011.

［10］　毛世瑞. 药剂学. 北京：人民卫生出版社，2019.

［11］　方亮，吕万良. 药剂学. 北京：人民卫生出版社，2016.

［12］　中华人民共和国药典（2020 版）. 北京：中国医药科技出版社，2015.

［13］　DailyMed. Moore medical non Aspirin- acetaminophen tablet, film coated. ［2021.7.8］. https://dailymed.nlm.nih.gov/dailymed/drugInfo.cfm?setid=d7b13248-397f-4cd4-9ad6-d042aa7e6e9c.

［14］　National Medical Products Administration. Provisions for Drug Insert Sheets and Labels. ［2006.3.15］. http://subsites.chinadaily.com.cn/nmpa/2019-07/25/c_390582.htm.

［15］　甘湘宁，周凤莲. 医药市场营销实务. 北京：中国医药科技出版社，2017，226-228.

［16］　Gartner. 18 Skills Every Salesperson Should Master. ［2019.8.12］. https://www.gartner.com/en/articles/18-skills-every-salesperson-should-master.

［17］　Pfizer. Medicine Safety Tips At Home. https://www.pfizer.com/products/medicine-safety/tips/at-home.

［18］　FDA. FDA Drug Safety Communication: Special storage and handling requirements must be followed for Pradaxa (dabigatran etexilate mesylate) capsules. ［2017.4.8］. https://www.fda.gov/drugs/drug-safety-and-availability/fda-drug-safety-communication-special-storage-and-handling-requirements-must-be-followed-pradaxa.